DEPARTMENT OF HEALTH & SOCIAL SECURITY

Prevention and health everybody's business

A reassessment of public and personal health

D0185034

London: Her Majesty's Stationery Office

ISBN 0 11 320188 5

Contents

Foreword

During the third quarter of this century our health services have passed through two main phases of development. The early years saw a concentration of effort directed to ensuring that the major specialties in hospital medicine were brought within reach of the population in every part of the country. More recently attention has focused on re-structuring the primary care services in order to foster closer collaboration not only between groups of doctors but also between them and other members of the domiciliary team.

The effects of these changes have already been far reaching. However, it is at least possible that in the absence of unforeseen and economical new methods of treatment, curative medicine may be increasingly subject to the law of diminishing returns.

Accordingly we believe that the time has come for a re-appraisal of the possibilities inherent in prevention. This is not so much a new initiative as a re-exploration of a well-tested, traditional approach.

Before re-organisation in 1974 the main statutory responsibility for prevention lay with the local authorities. As this consultative document makes plain, however, the preventive approach should permeate and inform all aspects of the health services. Moreover it is not restricted to the National Health Service since there are many activities in other fields, for example, in environmental health, food standards and the education and social services which have significant effects on the nation's health. The re-organised NHS, however, provides an improved administrative framework within which it is now possible to look at priorities more comprehensively and to plan the allocation of resources more effectively both at local and at national levels.

The aim of this booklet is to stimulate discussion on the possible contributions of prevention towards the solution of our health problems. It does not seek to be comprehensive but rather to draw attention to some general principles, to illustrate these by examples and to suggest how the prevention of disease and the promotion of health can best be advanced. It will be followed by further papers dealing more fully with specific issues.

Because of the pressures on resources of money and manpower in the health and other public services the opportunities for new developments in prevention will necessarily be limited in the near future. But the object of this document is not to recommend specific programmes but to start people thinking and talking about the place of prevention in the overall, longer term development of the health and related services. Thus members of National Health Service field authorities including members of Community and Local Health Councils need, in considering and planning the use of resources, to keep themselves informed about preventive measures and their potential so that they can ensure that full weight is given to their development. During the present period of economic restraint it is all the more essential that available resources are used to best effect, bearing in mind that not all preventive measures necessarily require additional, or massive resources. Much could be done by more effective deployment of existing staff and facilities; and much will depend on encouraging members of the public to make better use of the preventive services already available. We as a society are becoming increasingly aware of how much depends on the attitude and actions of the individual about his health. Prevention today is everybody's business.

BARBARA CASTLE
Secretary of State for Social Services

WILLIAM ROSS
Secretary of State for Scotland

JOHN MORRIS
Secretary of State for Wales

MERLYN REES
Secretary of State for Northern Ireland

CHAPTER I The background

Introduction

A century ago only six babies out of ten survived to adulthood, such were the ravages of disease, undernourishment, squalor and ignorance. The expectation of life at birth for a British boy born between 1871 and 1880 was 41 years, and for his sister 45, but if they survived the first hazardous year of life this expectation improved to 48 and 50 years. Today, this picture has been radically transformed. The reasons for this transformation are complex and, insofar as they are due to the practice of medicine itself, owe far more to preventive than to curative medicine. A great battle has been won and at first sight victory seems almost complete; but a second look shows a different picture. Most people can expect to live longer than in past generations but many still die prematurely or are, for many years of their life, dogged by avoidable ill health. The smoker's-cough (and worse), old people immobilised by deformed feet, and the health problems caused by over eating and under exercising are every day reminders of the continuing scope for prevention. We all need to be more aware of how we can help ourselves, our families and the community as a whole to avoid illnesses and their consequences. It is with these considerations in mind that this paper has been written.

This is essentially a consultative document intended to arouse discussion and invite comment. Its aim is to pose questions and offer a challenge to the health services and to those concerned with it both as providers and users. We need to interest individuals, communities and society as a whole in the idea that prevention is better than cure.

To move forward effectively with new developments in prevention we first need to know where we are and how we got here – the successes and mistakes that have been made in the past which will help to guide our way for the future. Accordingly the rest of this chapter examines in more detail the changes in life expectation and what has brought these about over the past 100 years. Chapter II will look at some success stories. However, when we come to Chapter III, which looks at the health problems facing us today, it will be seen that some are different in nature from those facing our forefathers a century ago since they are concerned with individual human behaviour or life-style rather than with the massive problems of environmental health and infectious disease. This is not to say that we can relax our guard against the infectious diseases – lest they should return to ravage an unguarded population; nor can we rest on the fact that many environmental health problems have disappeared – for they have often been replaced by new ones. The risk of infection from sewage is now virtually non-existent but there is an increasing need to scrutinise, for health hazards, the growing number of new chemical products which can affect the environment. Again, in the last half century, while the expectation of life at early ages in both sexes has continued to lengthen, this improvement has been much less marked in the older age groups, and especially among men. (Fig 1.1).[1]

Chapter IV looks at differences in mortality statistics and at the widely differing incidence of disease[2] between the United Kingdom and the other western nations, between regions within the United Kingdom itself, and between the various social classes. But is it an unalterable law of nature that the infant mortality rate in Scandinavian children should be lower than in British children or that it should be lower in the upper social classes among British children rather than in the less-favoured social classes? Following on from this, the later chapters examine some of the techniques used in prevention and consider certain new developments.

The above paragraphs set out what this paper is about. It is important also to realise what it is not concerned with. It is not intended as a definitive statement of government policy. Nor is it an examination of specific health issues in depth, though of course many are mentioned in order to illustrate the nature of present-day problems and the issues involved in overcoming them. It is the intention to follow-up this document with a series of more detailed papers covering such topics as smoking and alcoholism and examining the methods used in prevention.

---

[1] It has not been considered appropriate to provide detailed references to the many and varied statistics quoted in this paper and used to prepare the charts and graphs. The population, morbity and mortality statistics used however, have been obtained from the Office of Population, Censuses and Surveys (for England and Wales) and the General Register Offices of Scotland and Northern Ireland. The international statistics used have been obtained from the World Health Organisation's Statistics Annual.

[2] Throughout this paper the word 'disease' is used as a shorthand designation for 'disease, injury, disability and untimely death'.

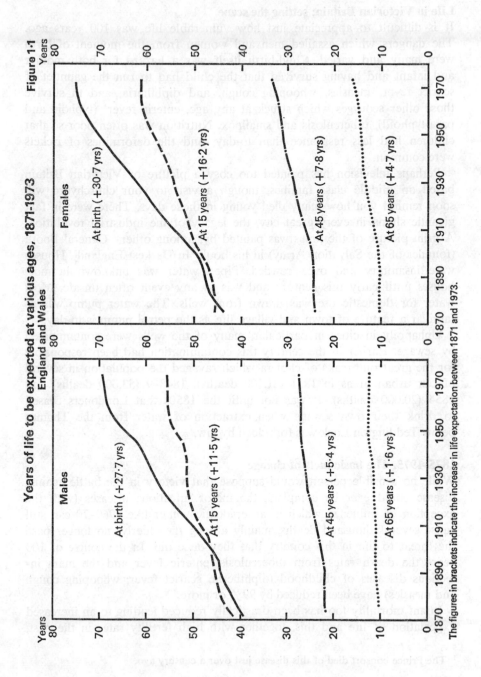

Figure 1·1

Years of life to be expected at various ages, 1871-1973
England and Wales

Males

At birth (+27·7 yrs)

At 15 years (+11·5 yrs)

At 45 years (+5·4 yrs)

At 65 years (+1·6 yrs)

Females

At birth (+30·7 yrs)

At 15 years (+16·2 yrs)

At 45 years (+7·8 yrs)

At 65 years (+4·7 yrs)

The figures in brackets indicate the increase in life expectation between 1871 and 1973.

Life in Victorian Britain: setting the scene

It is difficult to appreciate just how vulnerable life was 100 years ago. The dangers which assailed men and women from the moment of birth were many and varied. Child-birth itself was a hazard for both mother and infant and having survived that the child had to run the gauntlet of scarlet fever, measles, whooping cough, and diphtheria, and to survive those other scourges which struck at any age, enteric fever[1] (typhoid and para-typhoid), tuberculosis and smallpox. Nutrition was often poor so that children had less resistance than to-day, and the deformities of rickets were common.

Perhaps television has painted too cosy a picture of Victorian Britain based on middle class families, though a visit to your churchyard will soon remind you how many died young in those days. There were in fact gigantic slums in every great city, the legacy of the industrial revolution. A grim picture of the times was painted by, among others, General Booth (founder of the Salvation Army) in his book 'In Darkest England'. Houses were insanitary and over-crowded. Piped water was unknown in most houses until early this century and was in any event often unsafe. Most water for domestic use was drawn from wells. The water pump was as familiar a feature of town and village life as the petrol pump is to-day.

Unhappily in cities in particular, many of the wells were contaminated by sewage. Earlier in the century this contamination had been responsible for the great outbreaks of cholera which ravaged the population in several of our urban areas in 1831 (21,800 deaths), 1848-9 (53,000 deaths) and 1854 (20,000 deaths). It was not until the 1850s that Londoners ceased to drink their own sewage when extraction of water from the Thames below Teddington Lock was forbidden by law.

1875-1975. The basic facts of change

While no sensible person would suppose that victory in the battle against disease could ever be complete, the major infectious diseases (with the exception of influenza which in an epidemic winter like 1969-70 can still cause several thousand deaths, mainly among the elderly) no longer pose the threat to life in this country that they once did. In the course of 100 years the death rates from tuberculosis, enteric fever and the main infectious diseases of childhood (diphtheria, scarlet fever, whooping cough and measles) have been reduced by 99% or more.

Infant mortality too has been drastically reduced leading to an increased expectation of life and this, together with high fertility rates in the past,

---

[1] The Prince consort died of this disease just over a century ago.

Sex and age structure of the population

Figure 1·2

United Kingdom

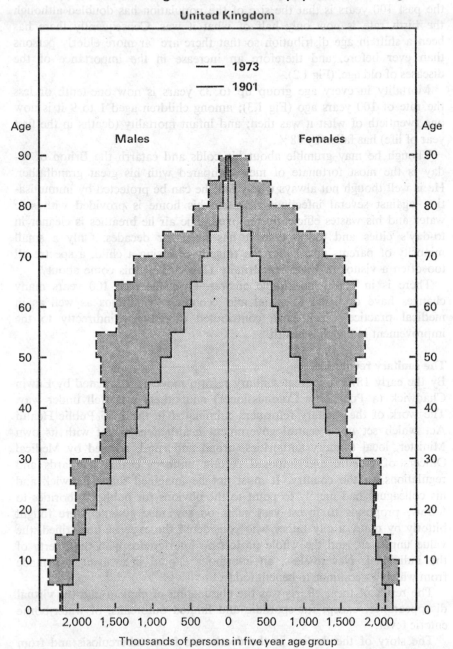

Thousands of persons in five year age group

have led to an enlarged population. Baldly stated what has happened in the past 100 years is that the size of the population has doubled although the birth rate is now only half of what it was. Consequently there has been a shift in age distribution so that there are far more elderly persons than ever before, and therefore an increase in the importance of the diseases of old age. (Fig 1.2).

Mortality in every age group up to 35 years is now one-tenth or less the rate of 100 years ago (Fig 1.3); among children aged 1 to 9 it is now one twentieth of what it was then; and infant mortality (deaths in the first year of life) has fallen by 88%.

Though he may grumble about his colds and catarrh the Briton of to-day is the most fortunate of men compared with his great grandfather. He is well though not always wisely fed; he can be protected by immunisation against several infectious diseases; his home is provided with safe water and his wastes efficiently removed. The air he breathes is cleaner in to-day's cities and towns than it has been for decades. Only a small minority of parents now suffer the tragedy of losing a child, a spectre all too often a visitor in Victorian Britain. How has all this come about?

There is in reality no simple answer. Over the past 100 years many changes have occurred in social and economic conditions as well as in medical practice which have contributed directly or indirectly to the improvement in people's health.

The sanitary revolution
By the early 1870s the great sanitary reform movement initiated by Edwin Chadwick (a Poor Law Commissioner) and others was well under way. The work of the sanitary reformers culminated in the 1875 Public Health Act which set up a central government health department with its own Minister, local sanitary authorities, urban and rural, advised by Medical Officers of Health, and imposed certain uniform health standards and regulations on the country. It must not be imagined that Chadwick and his colleagues had merely to point to the obvious for public authorities to follow; proposals to invest vast sums on sewerage systems were fought bitterly by many a city father who considered the expense unjustified, the value unproven, and the whole project an interference with the liberty of the individual. Nevertheless, an enormous capital investment was made from which we continue to benefit today.

The result of these efforts was the elimination of cholera and the virtual disappearance, except for sporadic and limited outbreaks, of water-borne enteric fever.

The story of the decline in the death rate from tuberculosis and from

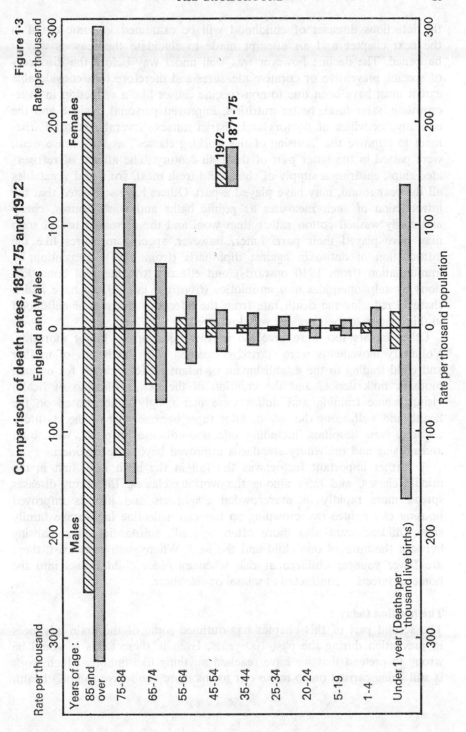

Figure 1·3

Comparison of death rates, 1871-75 and 1972
England and Wales

the infectious diseases of childhood will be examined in some detail in the next chapter and an attempt made to elucidate the reasons why it happened. The decline however was well under way before the discovery of specific preventive or curative measures and therefore to a considerable extent must have been due to non-specific causes like a reduction in over-crowding, safer food, better nutrition, improved personal hygiene and the educative activities of doctors and district nurses. Several Acts of Parliament to improve the 'housing of the working classes', as the phrase went, were passed in the latter part of the 19th century. The advent of refrigerated ships, ensuring a supply of cheap and fresh meat, fruit, and vegetables all the year round, may have played a part. Others have suggested that the introduction of such measures as public baths and wash houses, cheap and easily washed cotton rather than wool and the increased use of soap may have played their part. Later, however, specific measures like the introduction of antitoxin against diphtheria (from 1891), prevention by immunisation (from 1940 onwards) and effective treatment of complications by sulphonamides and antibiotics (from the late 1930s) have had a share in reducing the death rate from the infectious diseases of childhood in this country to their present very low levels.

Other factors too were involved in the reduction of infant mortality. Voluntary movements were started concerned with the health of mother and child leading to the establishment of infant clinics, schools for nursing mothers, milk depots and the creation of the new profession of health visitor whose training and duties were increasingly concentrated on the health and welfare of the infant; later these became part of the statutory services. New hospitals, including infectious disease hospitals, were built and nursing and midwifery standards improved beyond recognition.

A further important factor was the fall in the birth rate, first in the middle classes, and later among the working classes. Infectious diseases spread more rapidly in overcrowded conditions and just as improved housing can reduce overcrowding so too can a decline in average family size. Children were also more often 'spaced', substantial gaps elapsing between the birth of one child and the next. Where such gaps exist, there are fewer younger children at risk when an older child brings into the home an infection contracted at school or elsewhere.

The position today

The second part of this chapter has outlined some of the main advances in prevention during the past 100 years. Even in these fields it would be wrong to pretend that we have reached anything like finality. Much work is still being carried on to make our towns more conducive to good health by means of clear air legislation, steps to reduce road accidents and improvements in housing standards, to name but a few items. The work done in the last century by such pioneers as Lord Shaftesbury to improve and make safer the industrial environment, culminating in the first Factory Act and the appointment of factory inspectors is still being carried forward. Similarly with respect to infectious diseases the ground which has been gained must be held against attacks both by old diseases seeking to regain their superiority and by new infectious hazards. There are also fresh dangers such as the possible new forms of pollution from chemical, radiological and other sources. But many of the current major problems in prevention are related less to man's outside environment than to his own personal behaviour; what might be termed our life-style. For example the determination of many to smoke cigarettes in the face of the evidence that it is harmful to health and may well kill them; the failure to fasten seat belts in spite of the evidence that it saves lives; the reluctance to allow fluoride to be added to water supplies despite a proven benefit to dental health. These examples raise the question of whether man should be protected from himself either by legislation or by heavier taxation, for example of drink or tobacco? What is the role of Government in these matters? Is it largely the duty to educate, and to ensure that undue commercial pressures are not placed upon the individual and society? How far is the choice of the individual in these matters a free one and how can the individual be shown clearly the basis for the various options which are open to him so that he may make his choice with the greatest possible knowledge?

There are also the wider questions of how far we, as tax payers and rate payers, are prepared to pay in money and resources so that disease may be prevented. Advances in prevention must be paid for and the issue of costs and benefits is looked at in Chapter VII.

None of these issues is capable of a simple answer. The following chapters of this paper seek to bring out not only what remains to be done and the likely advantages from various possible developments, but also the difficulties, doubts and uncertainties which are to be found when considering the subject of prevention. For although prevention can be traced back to the health laws contained in the Laws of Moses, itself probably based on an earlier code, the picture is still far from complete and is nowadays changing more rapidly than ever. A vital object of this consultative document is therefore to persuade the reader, both as an individual and as a member of the community, that he needs to look at prevention afresh in the light of the needs of the fourth quarter of the twentieth century.

B

CHAPTER II Some success stories

Introduction

The long term consequences of some advances in prevention have been so dramatic that it is worth examining them in greater detail to see what lessons might be learned for today.

The major infectious scourges of the 19th century came in three broad groups comprising the mainly water borne diseases like cholera and enteric fever which affected all age groups; those infections, including diphtheria, measles, whooping cough and scarlet fever which affected mostly children; and those diseases like pulmonary tuberculosis and poliomyelitis which affected all age groups but young people in particular.

This chapter describes the decline in the mortality from these diseases and indeed the reduction in incidence of some to very low levels. It then examines the reduction in deaths of mothers in childbirth and concludes with an example of a form of screening successful in causing a sharp reduction in deaths from haemolytic disease of the newborn.

Cholera

As explained briefly in Chapter I, a series of cholera outbreaks occurred in the first half of the 19th century. While the capital was in the throes of its recurrent cholera epidemics a London doctor, John Snow, kept detailed records of patients contracting the disease, including their age, sex, dietary habits and so on. He was searching for a common factor in their daily lives and found it in the fact that each had drunk water, or consumed food or drink contaminated with water, from the Broad Street pump. The story goes that he became convinced of the cause of disease when he discovered that a cholera patient who had moved several miles from Soho to Highgate continued to get her water from Broad Street; the use of the pump was discontinued and the outbreak abated. The story may have been a little embellished with the passage of time but it is a good story and the basic facts are true.

The story illustrates first the value of statistical study to identify 'causes' of disease (part of the science of epidemiology); and second that it is not necessary to know all of the facts about a disease before taking preventive measures. The cholera vibrio, the germ which causes cholera, was not discovered for another thirty years but to know the 'cause' was in the water in the Broad Street pump was enough to allow effective action to be taken.

This principle exemplified by Snow that effective action can be taken on incomplete knowledge finds echoes in other fields of prevention. For example Percivall Pott incriminated coal-soot as a cause of skin cancer in 1775 but the chemical compound responsible in the soot was not identified until the 1930s. A century and a half separated James Lind's discovery that lime-juice prevented scurvy and the eventual isolation and synthesis of ascorbic acid (vitamin C).

Enteric fever (typhoid and paratyphoid)

Enteric fever was another major killer of the 19th century which was brought under control by improved sanitation. It is unlikely that it was realised at the time that enteric fever was also a water borne disease and in that sense Chadwick and his colleagues in providing safer water supplies and improved sewage disposal facilities 'builded better than they knew'. Certainly the reduction from decade to decade was spectacular as the quality of water supplies improved.

There was a slight check to progress after 1901, thought to be due to importation of the disease by soldiers returning from the Boer War but otherwise the decline has been swift and steady. (Fig 2.1).

Further impetus for the decline came from later measures to ensure the safety of milk, shell fish, ice cream and other foods through which enteric fever can also be spread. Today enteric fever in this country is relatively rare (some 200–250 cases a year in England and Wales) and in three out of four cases the infection is contracted abroad. There is always the danger of a carrier infecting food and, if that should have a wide distribution, a sizeable outbreak could occur. A high level of food hygiene together with appropriate checks on food handlers are the best safeguards against that happening.

Diphtheria

Together with measles and whooping cough, diphtheria was one of the most frequently fatal diseases of small children. Today it has been virtually eliminated and its decline ranks as one of the great triumphs of preventive medicine. It is now so rare that most doctors are unlikely to encounter it and it is difficult to appreciate the terror it held for parents until only about 35 years ago.

Diphtheria is an infection of the nose, mouth and throat which are

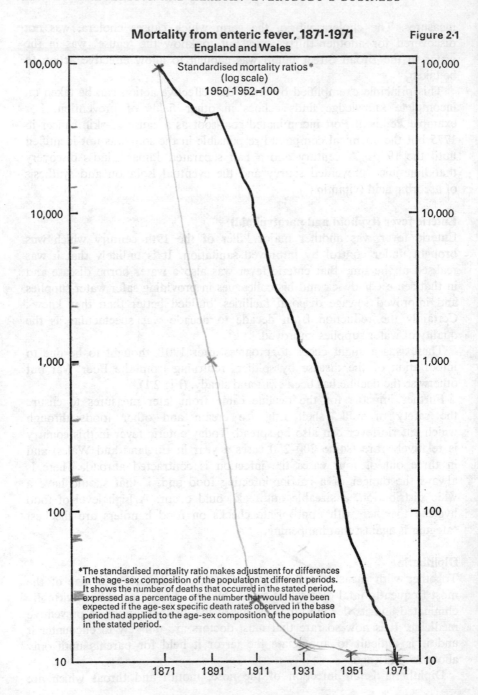

Mortality from enteric fever, 1871-1971
England and Wales

Figure 2·1

Standardised mortality ratios *
(log scale)
1950-1952=100

*The standardised mortality ratio makes adjustment for differences
in the age-sex composition of the population at different periods.
It shows the number of deaths that occurred in the stated period,
expressed as a percentage of the number that would have been
expected if the age-sex specific death rates observed in the base
period had applied to the age-sex composition of the population
in the stated period.

invaded by the growth of a distinctive grey membrane which constricts the air passages. Eventually a child, weakened by toxin produced by the diphtheria organism is liable to be literally suffocated. The death rate remained high in the 19th century but the development of an anti-toxin which could be given to the patient as soon as the disease was diagnosed played a large part in halving the death rate between 1900 and 1920. (Fig 2.2).

Even so between 1916 and 1925 there was an average of well over 50,000 cases a year and more than 4,000 children died annually. Between 1935 and 1942 deaths fell to an average of 2,780 but the number of cases remained at over 50,000. It was only after 1940, with the introduction of protection by active immunisation, that the incidence of diphtheria plummeted. Protection against diphtheria is now given to children as a matter of routine as part of the triple antigen immunisation (diphtheria, whooping cough and tetanus) with a booster on entry to school. In 1972–74[1] only seven cases were notified in Great Britain and there were no deaths.

Measles and whooping cough

More than 90% of all cases occur in children below the age of ten and the danger with both infections is that, in a small minority of cases complications such as pneumonia will develop and may be fatal. Measles vaccine has been generally available since 1968 but there is considerable concern that many mothers fail to take their children for measles vaccination with the result that epidemics still occur. Fewer than 70 per cent of children are vaccinated at present despite an incidence of 102,000 cases in England and Wales alone in the first six months of 1975.

One of the interesting facts about measles and whooping cough is that although specific treatment for complications was not available until the introduction of sulphonamide drugs in the 1930s, and prevention by vaccine in the late 1940s in the case of whooping cough, there was nevertheless a substantial fall in death rates from both diseases in the early decades of the century (Fig 2.3). Why this should be is a matter for speculation. There is no evidence that, up to World War Two, the incidence of either disease was declining. Fewer deaths therefore must have been due to the organism becoming less virulent or the child population becoming better able to withstand attack. The likelihood is that the multiple factors outlined in Chapter I, including better nutrition, less

[1] Throughout this paper the latest available statistics have been used. Wherever possible United Kingdom figures have been quoted but frequently because of lack of comparability or non-availability, Great Britain or England and Wales statistics have been used. The above are GB statistics.

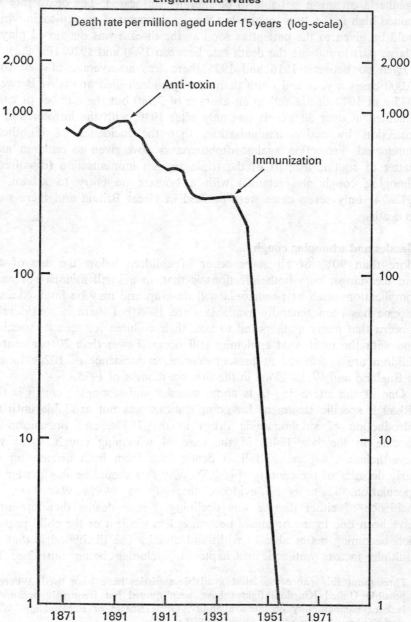

Childhood mortality from diphtheria, 1871-1971   Fig. 2·2
England and Wales

Death rate per million aged under 15 years (log-scale)

Anti-toxin

Immunization

Childhood mortality from measles and whooping-cough, 1871-1971
England and Wales

Fig.2·3

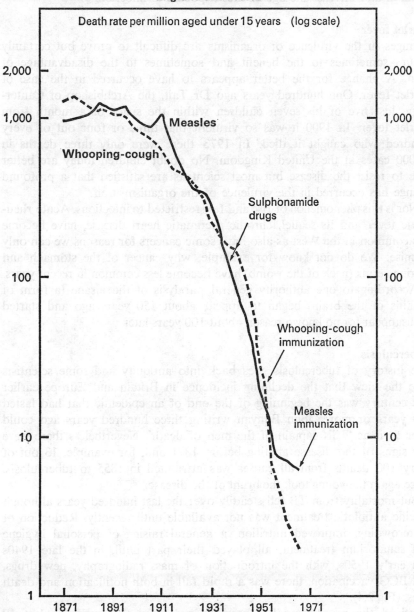

Death rate per million aged under 15 years   (log scale)

Measles

Whooping-cough

Sulphonamide drugs

Whooping-cough immunization

Measles immunization

overcrowding, smaller average family size and better housing, and wider 'spacing' of children all contributed to help reduce the vulnerability of children and increase the age of first exposure to infection.

Scarlet fever

Changes in the virulence of organisms are difficult to prove but certainly occur – sometimes to the benefit and sometimes to the disadvantage of man. A change for the better appears to have occurred in the case of scarlet fever. One hundred years ago Dr Tait, the Archbishop of Canterbury, lost five of his seven children within the space of a month from scarlet fever. In 1900 it was so virulent that three or four out of every hundred who caught it died. In 1973 there were only three deaths in 13,000 cases in the United Kingdom. No doubt children today are better able to resist the disease but most scientists are satisfied that a profound change has occurred in the virulence of the organism itself.

Nor is this phenomenon of rise and fall restricted to infections. Acute rheumatic fever and its sequel, chronic rheumatic heart disease, have become less common in the West as also have some cancers for reasons we can only surmise. We do not know for example, why cancer of the stomach and uterine cervix (neck of the womb) have become less common in recent years.

According to one authority general paralysis of the insane (a form of syphilis of the brain) began to appear about 150 years ago and started to disappear for no known reason about 100 years later.

Tuberculosis

The history of tuberculosis goes back into antiquity and some scientists take the view that the declining incidence in Britain and Europe earlier this century was the beginning of the end of an epidemic that had lasted 200 years or more. John Bunyan writing three hundred years ago could refer to it as 'This captain of the men of death'. Nevertheless there were few signs of the disease abating before 1871 and, for example, 13 out of every 100 deaths from all causes was attributed in 1855 to tuberculosis. Once again the young took the brunt of the disease.

But mortality from TB fell steadily over the last hundred years although specific antibiotic treatment was not available until recently. Reduction of overcrowding, improved nutrition, a general raising of personal hygiene and sanatorium treatment, all played their part until, in the late 1940s and early 1950s, with the introduction of mass radiography, new drugs, and BCG vaccination, there was a rapid fall in both notification and death rates. (Fig 2.4).

Indeed the programme has been so successful that over the last 10

Mortality from tuberculosis, 1871-1971   Figure 2·4

England and Wales

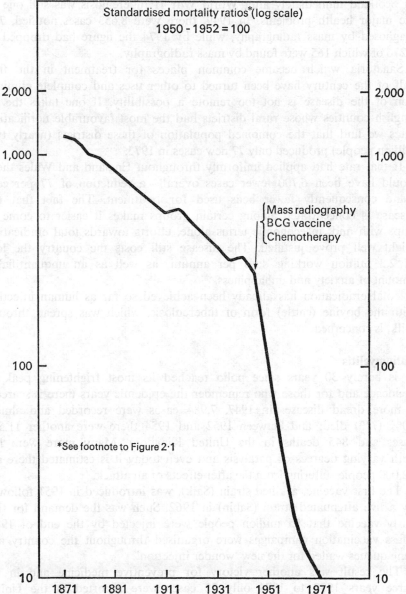

Standardised mortality ratios*(log scale)
1950 - 1952 = 100

Mass radiography
BCG vaccine
Chemotherapy

*See footnote to Figure 2·1

years or so the use of mass radiography has been almost completely discontinued. New cases are now largely confined to elderly men and groups such as immigrants who are particularly susceptible. (See page 36.) In Scotland immediately after World War II tuberculosis was still one of the major health problems. In 1949, there were 8,653 cases notified, 734 diagnosed by mass radiography, while by 1974 the figure had dropped to 1,276 of which 165 were found by mass radiography.

Sanatoria which became common places for treatment in the first half of the century have been turned to other uses and complete elimination of the disease is not too remote a possibility. If one takes the 12 English counties whose rural districts had the most favourable notification rates we find that the combined population of these districts (nearly two million people) produced only 77 new cases in 1973.

If that rate had applied uniformly throughout England and Wales there would have been 6,700 fewer cases overall – a reduction of 77 per cent – and consequently fewer beds used for treatment. The fact that the disease is concentrated among certain groups makes it easier to come to grips with and, in economic terms alone, efforts towards total eradication might well prove justified. The disease still costs the country the loss of 2.3 million working days per annum, as well as an unquantifiable amount of anxiety and unhappiness.

Total eradication has already been achieved so far as human infection with the bovine (cattle) form of tuberculosis, which was spread through milk, is concerned.

Poliomyelitis

It is barely 30 years since polio reached its most frightening peak of incidence and for those who remember the epidemic years there is scarcely a more dread disease. In 1947, 7,984 cases were recorded and almost 10% (713) died; and between 1952 and 1954 there were another 11,500 cases and 845 deaths in the United Kingdom. Many more were left with varying degrees of paralysis and even today it is estimated there are 12,000 people suffering from the after effects of an attack.

The first vaccine, a killed strain (Salk), was introduced in 1957 followed by a live attenuated strain (Sabin) in 1962. Such was the demand for that early vaccine that 15 million people were injected by the end of 1960. Mass vaccination campaigns were organised throughout the country and long queues waited for the new 'wonder injection'.

The result was another victory for preventive medicine and in the three years 1972 to 1974 only 22 cases were reported in the United Kingdom, with no deaths. Because poliomyelitis still lingers on in some countries, and the virus may be imported, vaccination is still important. Indeed now that smallpox – the earliest disease for which vaccination became possible – has reached such a stage of control that the World Health Organisation can talk realistically about its imminent extinction, polio vaccination is more important than smallpox vaccination for travellers abroad.

Public memory is short and the worrying aspect about the polio vaccination programme is that, incredibly, one child in three is now not being taken for vaccination. This is despite the fact that there is no measure less troublesome or less dangerous for the child or more convenient for the mother.

Maternal mortality

The quite astonishing reduction in deaths of mothers during pregnancy and childbirth can most fairly be classed a victory for 'the system', a quite different aspect of prevention from those which we have witnessed so far in this chapter. A planned attack, which included higher professional standards among doctors and midwives combined with effective use of the legislative and administrative machinery and the use of epidemiological techniques, was the key. Between 1928 and 1935 maternal mortality varied from 40 to 45 deaths for every 10,000 pregnancies. That was an average of about 2,500 deaths in any single year. This tragic and avoidable waste of life stirred the conscience of the nation and in the early 1930s a national drive was launched and sustained aimed at safer motherhood.

The establishment of the Royal College of Obstetricians and Gynaecologists was an important feature of this period as was the Midwives Act of 1936; midwives were given better training; better arrangements were made for the care of pregnant women and later for their confinement, where possible, in hospital; and more hospital beds under specialist supervision were provided as quickly as resources allowed.

A powerful political commitment sustained the momentum of the campaign which happily coincided with an improvement of nutrition during pregnancy and important technical advances; in the early detection and control of high blood pressure in pregnancy; in anaesthesia and blood transfusion; and the control of puerperal fever, the dreaded 'blood poisoning' once so common in women after childbirth.

It has also been said that the 'efficiency' of mothers in pregnancy and childbirth is related to their life-long nutrition. As has been stated nutritional standards had been rising and this too must have had an effect.

The impetus of the 1930s was not allowed to dissipate and once the

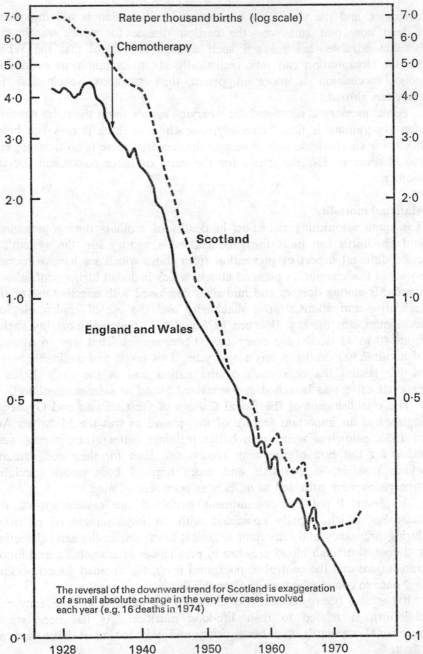

Maternal mortality, 1928-1974

Figure 2·5

Scotland, England and Wales

Rate per thousand births (log scale)

Chemotherapy

Scotland

England and Wales

The reversal of the downward trend for Scotland is exaggeration
of a small absolute change in the very few cases involved
each year (e.g. 16 deaths in 1974)

Northern Ireland cannot be included in this diagram as still-births were not reported
until 1961. The maternal mortality rate per 1,000 live-births was, for Northern
Ireland however, 5.2 per 1,000 in 1928 and 0.2 per 1,000 in 1974.

administrative machinery was in being, it was possible to take rapid steps in the light of clinical advances. A valuable technique, introduced nationally in 1952, was impartial expert examination of the facts surrounding each maternal death to establish whether and if so why 'the system' had failed. This was an early example of what has become known as medical audit.

The net result is that maternal deaths in England and Wales occur now in only one out of every 10,000 pregnancies (Fig 2.5). Satisfactory though that is there is evidence that it could be improved still further because, unfortunately, some maternal deaths with 'avoidable' factors still occur. Figure 2.5 also shows the decline in maternal mortality in Scotland; research carried out in Aberdeen identified pregnant women 'at special risk' so that special arrangements for their care and confinement, could be made. The effects of this work were felt far beyond Aberdeen. This shows how the improved use of existing resources can be as important as the provision of new resources.

Haemolytic disease of the newborn
Chapter VI will discuss at length the considerations which arise when making a decision on whether to adopt a new 'screening' procedure. (Screening involves examination of apparently healthy people to detect those who are likely to develop a disease or who may have already done so but at an early stage). The idea is attractive but as will be shown there are pitfalls. However some forms of screening have been very successful, for example in its time mass radiography of the chest to detect pulmonary tuberculosis. Another successful form of screening is designed to detect the likelihood of and prevent, haemolytic disease of the newborn.

The story is fascinating. For many years doctors have been familiar with haemolytic disease of the newborn. Sometimes the condition is so severe as to cause stillbirth. In less severe cases the infant is born alive but anaemic, and often severely jaundiced. Death may follow but even if the infant survives he may be left brain-damaged, and often deaf.

As is well known everyone belongs to one of four main blood groups, namely A, B, AB and O. In 1941 it was discovered that people can also be classed into one of two other blood groups, namely rhesus positive or rhesus negative (87% and 13% respectively in Europeans). Haemolytic disease of the newborn can arise when a rhesus negative mother becomes pregnant by a rhesus positive father and the baby is rhesus positive. Exceptionally (and in only a small proportion of such pregnancies) some of the infant's red blood cells may leak from its blood circulation into the mother's blood. Over a period of months these foetal red blood cells cause the mother to produce a protective substance called antibody to destroy them. In a subsequent pregnancy, this protective antibody can cross over to the foetal circulation and destroy foetal red blood cells thus causing haemolytic disease of the newborn.

Soon after the discovery of the rhesus factor, a test for rhesus antibodies in pregnant women was developed, as well as a test for antibodies in the baby's circulation at birth. Thereafter screening tests for antibodies in rhesus negative mothers and their infants became routine. Treatment comprised induction of birth in the face of a rise in antibody level in the mother's blood, provided the foetus was viable (capable of independent existence). If the newborn infant was severely affected replacement transfusion could be performed and the infant's blood containing maternal antibody and destroyed red blood cells replaced with normal blood. In recent years a new technique has been perfected for preventing the condition developing in most cases by identifying all rhesus negative women and, subsequent to first delivery, or abortion, injecting a tiny amount of antibody which immediately destroys any foetal red blood cells which may have leaked into the maternal circulation. Large amounts of antibody then do not develop.

The essential factors then are screening all pregnant women to identify the rhesus negative, injection to prevent the condition developing in most cases; screening all rhesus negative women in every subsequent pregnancy to detect the odd person who nevertheless become sensitised; and screening their infants to make assurance doubly certain.

As a result of the unravelling of this story and the measures taken deaths of live-born infants from this disease have fallen (England and Wales) from 505 in 1951 to 105 in 1973. Statistics for still births are available only for recent years; they show a fall between 1968 and 1972 from 473 to 258. (Note that a small number of deaths is due to other rare blood group incompatibilities). There is, however, further room for improvement, and almost complete elimination of the disease due to rhesus incompatability is possible.

These two stories, of the reduction in maternal mortality and in deaths from haemolytic disease of the newborn provide examples of effective prevention which has been achieved in fields other than the infectious diseases.

CHAPTER III Some problems of today and tomorrow

The broad categories of disease

In Britain to-day the spectrum of health problems contains three principal categories relevant to this chapter. In one group are the problems which are in one sense the consequence of successful prevention in past decades, notably the diseases and disabilities associated with old age, resulting from the enormous growth in the proportion of the population who are aged.

A second group includes those diseases the cause of which and the solution to which can be laid at the door of man's behaviour. Radical alterations in attitudes, social conventions and behaviour are giving rise to new health problems or to old problems in a new form. Affluence is not an unqualified boon and while it has certainly enabled us to avoid some diseases, for example those due to nutritional deficiency, it has opened the door to others arising, for instance, from unwise behaviour and over-indulgence in one form or another.

Third comes a group of hazards related to our changing environment. Technological developments in transport and communications, in industry, and in the production and marketing of food, are having an effect for better or worse on people's health, whilst the physical environment itself is undergoing changes in a number of other relevant ways.

Before considering these three main categories, it will be of interest to look at the size of the problems involved, both as they concern sickness and death.

Illness today

CAUSES OF DEATH

The most important causes of death in this country today are heart disease, cancer and stroke, in that order and together these account in England and Wales for 66% of all mortality. These are diseases that strike heavily with advancing age and it is important to appreciate that 72 per cent of all deaths occur at ages from 65 years and onwards.

Most of the deaths that happen in the first year occur before the end of the first week, the main causes being immaturity, birth injury and congenital abnormalities. For the rest of the first year respiratory diseases, congenital abnormalities, 'sudden' deaths, infectious diseases and accidents, are the main causes in order of importance. Between the ages of 1 and 14 years the number of deaths is fortunately small and now accidents take first place with cancers, congenital abnormalities and respiratory diseases being responsible for most of the remaining deaths.

During the productive years (15 to 64) the position differs among males and females. For men the most important single cause by far is ischaemic heart disease ('coronaries') and indeed this one cause is responsible for more years of productive life lost than any other single disease. Among women in this age range cancers are the leading cause of death with breast cancer the most important single cancer. Cancer is also a major killer among men under 65 with lung cancer of all the cancers far and away the biggest threat to life. Strokes are numerically important in both sexes with accidents and bronchitis being the other leading causes for males. By comparison, such conditions as tuberculosis, peptic ulcer, appendicitis, intestinal obstruction and hernia – all diseases for which effective treatment is available – are relatively trivial as causes of death of adults under the age of 65 years. Some of the important features of the pattern of mortality at different ages are well illustrated in Figure 3.1.

Table 3.1 Trends in death rates at ages 45–64 years by causes in the United Kingdom, 1963–1973.

Falling	Rising
Tuberculosis	Cancer of lung (females)
Cancer of stomach	Ischaemic heart disease
Hypertensive disease	
Bronchitis	
*Cancer of lung (males)	
*Cerebrovascular disease	
Suicide	

* Not Northern Ireland

Deaths in age groups indicating the main causes, 1972 Fig. 3·1

United Kingdom

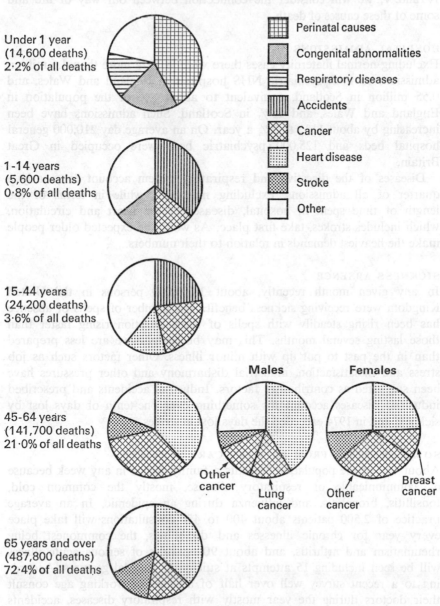

Under 1 year
(14,600 deaths)
2·2% of all deaths

1-14 years
(5,600 deaths)
0·8% of all deaths

15-44 years
(24,200 deaths)
3·6% of all deaths

45-64 years
(141,700 deaths)
21·0% of all deaths

65 years and over
(487,800 deaths)
72·4% of all deaths

Perinatal causes

Congenital abnormalities

Respiratory diseases

Accidents

Cancer

Heart disease

Stroke

Other

Males

Females

Other cancer

Lung cancer

Other cancer

Breast cancer

a

Table 3.1 lists the diseases with falling or rising death rates in middle life during the recent years. Later in this Chapter and again in Chapters IV and V, we will consider the connection between our way of life and some of these causes of death.

HOSPITAL ADMISSIONS
Excluding normal maternity cases there were in 1972 more than 4.6 million admissions to non-psychiatric NHS hospitals in England and Wales, and 0.55 million in Scotland, equivalent to about 8% of the population in England and Wales, and 13% in Scotland. Such admissions have been increasing by about $1\frac{1}{2}$% to 2% a year. On an average day 210,000 general hospital beds and 125,000 psychiatric beds were occupied in Great Britain.

Diseases of the digestive and respiratory system account for nearly a quarter of all admissions, excluding maternity, while in terms of the length of time spent in hospital, diseases of the heart and circulation, which includes strokes, take first place. As would be expected older people make the heaviest demands in relation to their numbers.

SICKNESS ABSENCE
In any given month recently, about 1,000,000 persons in the United Kingdom were receiving sickness benefit. The number of spells of absence has been rising steadily with spells of short duration rising faster than those lasting several months. This may be because we are less prepared than in the past to put up with minor illness. Other factors such as job stress and dissatisfaction, industrial disharmony and other pressures have been suggested as contributory factors. Industrial accidents and prescribed industrial diseases account for something over one-tenth of days lost by sickness and in 1974 exceeded the days lost in strikes.

SOME EVIDENCE FROM PRIMARY CARE SERVICES
About 1% of the population consults a family doctor in any week because of communicable or respiratory disease, mostly the common cold, tonsillitis, bronchitis, and influenza during an epidemic. In an average practice of 2,500 patients about 400 to 450 consultations will take place every year for chronic illnesses and disabilities, the commonest being rheumatism and arthritis, and about 90 episodes of serious acute illness will be seen including 15 attempts at suicide or suicidal gestures. According to a recent survey well over half of all men of working age consult their doctors during the year mostly with respiratory diseases, accidents (sprains, cuts, etc), skin conditions, lumbago, rheumatism, arthritis and

mental and nervous conditions, in that order. There will also be about 200 consultations with a primary preventive purpose, for example immunisation, each year in an average practice. Nurses, health visitors and domiciliary midwives attached to general practice form an increasingly important element in primary health care.

The most prevalent disease of all is dental caries. More will be said about teeth, and in particular about fluoride, when we come to discuss the practicalities of prevention in Chapter v. Suffice to say the number of courses of dental treatment (27 million in 1973) is equivalent to nearly half the population; about 9,000,000 teeth are extracted and 36,000,000 filled in Great Britain every year. A high proportion of the population have no natural teeth by middle age, having to rely on dentures, and even among children the incidence of dental caries is appalling.

A detailed survey in one area of Wales recently showed that the average 5 year old child already had 6.4 damaged teeth and the average 15 year old had 11.4 teeth affected. In another country-wide survey 7 out of 10 children entering school had dental decay and 4 out of 5 eight year olds had actively decaying teeth requiring treatment.

Demographic changes

Profound changes in the age and sex constitution of the population this century have had far reaching consequences for the nature of health problems to-day. The population of the United Kingdom has increased this century from 38,000,000 to 56,000,000 and the age structure has altered significantly (see figure 1.2). In 1901 people of retirement age (males aged 65 and females aged 60 and over) accounted for only 6% of the population. By 1971 the proportion had risen to 16%.

Of recent years the most remarkable demographic feature has been the rapid decline in the number of births. Birth rates rise and fall for a variety of reasons, but there can be no doubt that the introduction of new family planning techniques, the spread of knowledge about them, and the widespread acceptability of open discussion about family planning have produced a better-informed public well able to control their fertility if they choose to do so. Indeed, at a time when the age of marriage has been falling, the acceptability of contraception and improvements in contraceptive practice (together with changes consequent on abortion legislation) must have played some part in the fall in the number of births by 172,000 (in England and Wales) between 1964 and 1974, a reduction of 20% in a decade.

In particular there are now fewer births to older mothers and women who might otherwise have had larger families. One important side effect both of the total reduction of births and the reduction in births to older mothers is that fewer infants are now born with Down's Syndrome (mongolism) which is known to be more common among babies born to mothers reproducing late in life. It has been calculated that compared with 1964 there were 440 (26%) fewer affected infants born in 1973.

A further demographic change of some significance to health, is migration both into and within the country. Whenever people migrate either from one continent to another or from the countryside to the city, health problems are likely to arise. Close to half a million immigrants from the New Commonwealth (including Pakistan) entered this country in the past ten years. Some 460,000 born on the Indian sub-continent and another 300,000 born in the West Indies were enumerated at the 1971 Census. In addition that census revealed 700,000 of Irish origin and another 1,000,000 from a variety of other countries.

Understandably immigrants, especially those who do not share our language or cultural background, tend to congregate in the same areas. Greater London and the West Midlands have attracted the largest numbers. Only too often immigrants live, for a time at least, in undesirably over-crowded conditions. Some immigrant groups present unique medical problems. For example, there are certain forms of blood disorder which affect Cypriots and others of Eastern Mediterranean origin. But tuberculosis and rickets are two other diseases which, though not confined to immigrants, are prevalent among them. Immigrants are inevitably subject to psycho-social strains in adapting to their new surroundings and problems of mental health and disorders of behaviour can result particularly among children and adolescents.

Health problems of the aged
The increased longevity of the population is strikingly reflected in the median age of death. In Britain, in 1973, half of all deaths of men occurred at the age of 70 or over. Among women it was 76 or over. Fifty years ago the median age of death was only 55 for men and 60 for women. About 6½ million people in the United Kingdom are now aged 65 to 74 and another 2.7 million are 75 and over. Most (over 90%) are at present able to live in their own homes, many under the care of the district nurse or health visitor and assisted by home helps. These are the people who were among the first to benefit from improvement in health since the turn of the century, and the bulge in their numbers is clearly shown in figure 1.2.

The latest estimates suggest that in 25 years time the number over 75 years of age will increase by another 700,000 in England and Wales alone, and if the demands people of this age make on institutional beds continue at the present rate, an additional 65,000 places will be needed, comprising 9,000 in psychiatric hospitals, 22,000 in other hospitals and 34,000 in local authority accommodation. This raises formidable logistic problems which, coming at a time of financial restraint, may require a re-allocation of resources or a re-consideration of alternative solutions. An increasing number of old people inevitably means more cases of disability and more chronic degenerative disease. What is less readily recognised is the problem of isolation among the old. In Britain at the time of the 1971 census 144,000 men and 646,000 women aged 75 and over were living alone.

It is self evident that the scope for reducing overall mortality among the elderly is limited and some have questioned the morality of devoting large resources to seeking to extend their lives for what must inevitably be relatively short periods of time, especially when the quality of that extended life may sometimes be open to question not least by those affected. By comparison, even small reductions in mortality among the young are clearly worth striving for since more years of life will be saved than by reductions, even large ones, at older ages. It has been calculated that, for England and Wales, if all deaths during the productive years (15 to 64) were avoided the added years of life would amount to 592 years for every 10,000 men and 350 years for every 10,000 women.

We do not have comprehensive data on the amount of disability among the aged, but defects of sight, hearing, and mobility become increasingly common with advancing years. Registration is known to be incomplete, but about 14,000 new cases of blindness are registered every year in Great Britain, the most important causes being senile degenerative disorders, cataract, and glaucoma. It is estimated that a quarter of all people of 65 and over suffer from a significant degree of deafness and about a million people of all ages in this country use a hearing aid. To maintain their mobility, and in many cases their independence, large numbers of people of 65 and over need chiropody treatment (more than a million people of 65 and over receive National Health Service chiropody treatment every year).

Another problem liable to arise among the isolated elderly is nutritional deficiency. The reasons include immobility, inadequate management of money or the co-existence of other serious diseases and obviously a proportion of these cases are preventable. Since there are about 2.7 million people aged 75 and over in Britain, including 1.75 million single or widowed, if even a small proportion of them are affected, this would represent a large number of cases of preventable disease.

Thinning of the bones (osteoporosis) is a common finding in old people, affecting particularly old women, and may explain the high frequency of fracture of the wrist, the hip, and the spine among them. Research is at present being pursued to test various theories; one has it that the condition is caused by lack of vitamin D, another by reduced secretion of sex hormones after the menopause. Should it be possible to unravel the cause or causes and prevent this condition, the benefits in terms of releasing hospital beds could be substantial.

Behaviour and health

Perhaps the most difficult diseases to prevent are those which depend on individual behaviour. The role of Government here is a complex one, but Government already plays a part by means of fiscal (taxation) and legal controls on the manufacture, sale (or prohibition from sale) and on the promotion of certain products like alcohol, tobacco and drugs, and subsidises education relating to the use and misuse of such products. To a large extent though, it is clear that the weight of responsibility for his own state of health lies on the shoulders of the individual himself. The smoking related diseases, alcoholism and other drug dependencies, obesity and its consequences, and the sexually transmitted diseases are among the preventable problems of our time and in relation to all of these the individual must choose for himself.

SMOKING AND HEALTH

Although cigarette smoking among men has tended to decline steadily in recent years there is no evidence of such a decline among women. Between 1961 and 1973 the proportion of adult men who smoke manufactured cigarettes fell from 59% to 49%. Among women it remained much the same at 43%. However, the habit is certainly more common among women to-day than it was 30 or more years ago. Some other trends of importance have emerged in recent years. One is the encouraging decline in smoking among the professional classes; at the same time there has been a worrying increase among the wives of unskilled men. Another trend is that although the percentage of cigarette smokers in the adult population has fallen, those who continued to smoke were, in the early 1970's, smoking more. The most important diseases known to be caused or exacerbated by smoking are lung cancer, chronic bronchitis, and coronary heart disease. Many men in middle age are nowadays being called upon to pay again, and in a different currency, for the cigarettes they have smoked since their youth. It can be safely predicted that the incidence of these diseases among women will continue to rise so long as their smoking also continues to increase.

In Great Britain there has in fact been a slight fall in the death rate of men from lung cancer, but a sharp increase at ages 45 to 64 among women. Mortality from ischaemic heart disease (at ages 45 to 64) increased by 14% among men and by 20% among women in the 10 years to 1973.

Bronchitis by contrast has shown a declining trend in mortality and at ages 45 to 64 deaths among men in England and Wales have fallen from 123 per 100,000 in 1963 to 70 per 100,000 in 1973. The death rate of women in the same age group has fallen at a much slower rate. Trends in Scotland and Northern Ireland are similar. The most likely explanation for the decline is the steady extension of control of air pollution through the Clean Air Act, 1956, and equivalent Northern Ireland legislation.

ALCOHOLISM

A widespread and serious form of dependence in this country is alcoholism. Definitions vary and consequently so do estimates of prevalence, but it has been estimated that there may be as many as 500,000 people with a serious drink problem in England and Wales and proportionately more in Scotland where the problem is acknowledged to be of more serious dimensions. The problem is of course medico-social and extends beyond the affected individual to include family, friends and fellow employees. Convictions for offences in which alcohol is implicated have risen (though this may reflect legal changes and police policy) as have admissions to hospitals for treatment of alcoholism and alcoholic psychosis. The increase in such admissions between 1959 and 1973, from 2,000 to 11,500 in England and Wales, from just over 900 to 5,000 in Scotland, and from 900 to 1,500 in Northern Ireland between 1962 and 1973 shows the heavier work load on psychiatric services from treating these conditions. These admissions reflect service provisions, policies and attitudes, both of the treater and the treated and show wide variations between different parts of the United Kingdom. The strain on general hospital services of treating intoxicated patients is illustrated by the experience of the Western Infirmary in Glasgow. Two-thirds of men and a third of women admitted to that hospital for treatment for self poisoning or head injuries are found to have alcohol in the blood, and with mean blood alcohol concentrations above 100 mg per 100 ml, well in excess of the legal limit for drivers.

Cirrhosis of the liver is not as yet a major cause of death despite the level of alcoholism (there were 1,804 deaths in England and Wales in 1973) but the overall death rate from this disease has risen from 28 to 37 per million between 1963 and 1973. Men and women have similar rates and for both sexes the rise has been comparable. What seems likely is that at least some of the increase in drinking is the result of greater affluence. Twenty-five years ago a bottle of whisky cost 45% of the average man's weekly disposable income. To-day it costs less than 20% and consumption per head has quadrupled in the last quarter century.

MISUSE OF DRUGS

By comparison narcotic addiction is numerically a relatively minor problem. The number of narcotic addicts in Great Britain known to the Home Office as receiving treatment is about 2,000. Some claim that increasing reliance on tranquillisers, anti-depressants and hypnotics is a form of drug addiction. There were 46.6 million prescriptions for such drugs issued by general practitioners in 1973 in England, and their use has increased in the last ten years.

A related cause of hospital admission which has increased in recent years is self poisoning, mainly among young women. It is the commonest cause of admission of such women to acute medical wards. No matter whether these are cries for help or serious attempts at suicide there is undeniably an epidemic of self poisoning which shows no sign of abating.

The appetite of some sections of the media for sensational medical stories, 'wonder drugs', new operations and so on should not be ignored. This may have helped to foster the idea that medicine to-day can offer a 'pill for every ill'. It is of course a snare and a delusion but one that the health professions themselves have not always done all that they might to rectify.

THE USE OF LEISURE

Whether the increase in leisure (and the great majority of workers in Britain are now entitled to three or more weeks paid holiday a year) and the use that is made of it have served to promote better health is a moot point. It is estimated that 93% of homes in the United Kingdom have a television set and the average adult now spends more time watching television than in any other activity apart from sleep and work. The mechanisation of industry, the spread of car ownership and of labour saving devices in the home are other factors resulting in less call for strenuous muscular effort. Some experts, in this country and abroad, consider lack of exercise as one of the besetting sins of modern man which is having an adverse effect on his health.

NUTRITION

The national diet has changed gradually over many decades. Protein intake has varied comparatively little, but certain foods, notably bread, cereals, and potatoes are not as popular as they used to be. Sugar, which supplies no vitamins, minerals, or other essential nutrients, and fat, provide an increasing share of the total energy of the average diet. While an individual with a relatively high total energy intake may derive sufficient essential nutrients, a person with a lower energy requirement taking a badly balanced diet may be close to the margin of safety. The relevance of these changes to causation of coronary heart disease has been the subject of much controversy and both increased sugar intake and the increased intake of certain fats have been blamed as contributory factors. Whether either or both have a direct effect they could act simply by increasing the tendency to obesity, itself imposing a strain on the heart. But the national diet has improved in many respects; it has long been compulsory to fortify flour with vitamins, iron and calcium, and the provision of school meals and milk have also been important health-promoting measures.

THE SEXUAL REVOLUTION

There can be little doubt that we have been and are passing through a period when the role of women in society is changing. There is an increasing demand for greater equality of opportunity and for greater self-fulfilment and this is reflected in behaviour, including health related behaviour. We have noted that to some extent the smoking habits of women have approximated more closely to those of men and the same may be true for alcohol. There is also good evidence of changes in sexual attitudes among younger women. It so happens that these changes have occurred at the same time as advances in contraception, although there is also evidence that the safeguards against pregnancy offered by contraception are by no means always used. However the availability of legal abortion in certain circumstances since 1968 has served in some measure as a counter to contraceptive failure.

Like all scientific advances and social changes there have been benefits and disadvantages. Most people probably regard the retreat from the Victorian attitudes to sex which persisted until quite recently as an advance. Sexual problems, often due simply to ignorance, can cause great distress within marriage and discussion with a skilled adviser is no longer considered taboo, but indeed is being increasingly sought. At the same time sex before marriage seems increasingly common.

The result of sexual experience without efficient contraception in the unmarried is reflected in the incidence of pregnancy (itself in turn recorded reasonably accurately as abortions, illegitimate births and births legitimated by marriage). The incidence of illegal abortion is of course unknown. But what seems to have happened since 1968 is that there was an initial rise in the total of recorded extra-marital conceptions at all ages, that this steadied off after 1971, fell in young women of 20 and over but is still increasing in school girls under 16 (though the total involved is small in proportion to the total number of school girls).

Judging by the annual returns of the special clinics dealing with sexually transmitted diseases the number of cases seen has increased more than three-fold between 1959 and 1974. To some extent this increase undoubtedly reflects an increased willingness on the part of those infected – or who fear they may have been infected – to seek medical aid from these clinics. Additionally over the last 15 years there has been an increasing tendency to refer patients to the special clinics who would previously have been treated elsewhere, but it seems likely too that the increase is in part due to an increase in casual sexual encounters. (It has been said that the risk of disease is in inverse proportion to the length of time the partners have been known to each other – the shorter the time the greater the risk). The number of new cases of gonorrhoea has also been rising up to about four years ago, since when the numbers have not changed much. This may be a hopeful sign that the services concerned with the control of sexually transmitted diseases, particularly the tracing of sexual contacts of affected persons, are operating with increasing effect.

The physical environment and disease
In some respects our environment today is healthier than it has ever been. Air pollution has been brought under control over large populous areas by virtue of the Clean Air Act 1956. Although major problems persist in certain parts of the country and much could be done to meet the special needs of the elderly, housing has improved with an increasing provision of the basic amenities and the elimination of gross overcrowding.

In other respects the environmental position is more problematical. Road traffic expressed as passenger miles per annum approximately doubled from 1961 to 1974 with the number of vehicles increasing by 82%. Road deaths in Britain increased from 6,900 in 1961 to a peak of 8,000 in 1965, but by 1974, partly as a result of the fuel crisis, they had returned to 6,900. Serious injuries increased from 85,000 to almost 100,000 in the same period, but fell back to 82,000 in 1974.

Not all environmental hazards are necessarily fatal and there is increasing concern at the adverse effects of less dramatic irritants. Noise was made the subject of a code of practice in industry for the first time in

1972. Deafness associated with occupation, for example in boiler-makers and jute-weavers has been known for many years. Attention is turning now however to the mental as well as the physical effects of excessive noise. Chemical pollution of the environment is also attracting considerable attention, particularly where there is a risk of increased intake of heavy metals (especially lead) in children. A constant stream of new chemicals is finding uses in industry or in and around the home, with a possibility that any one of them may prove in the long term to be harmful.

CHAPTER IV The scope for prevention

Without Contraries is no Progression – William Blake

Introduction

The fact that one group of the population is less healthy than another group either in another part of Britain, in another social class, or in another country presents both a puzzle and a challenge to preventive medicine. It is a puzzle because the explanations for such differences are often obscure and a challenge because the fact that a difference exists at all suggests that there may be potential scope for improvement.

It has been argued, for example, that on a global basis, 85% of all cancers have environmental causes and are therefore potentially preventable, since that is the sum of the cancers that would not arise if the lowest known rate of occurrence of each separate type of cancer were to apply everywhere in the world.

When comparing countries it would clearly be preferable to study the prevalence of disease in the different populations concerned, but such information is not always available and we are therefore usually obliged to use death rate statistics which are published by the World Health Organisation for many countries and which can be more confidently compared.

General mortality – a comparison with Sweden

Sweden has long enjoyed one of the best health records of any country and it is salutary to see how the Swedish mortality experience compares with that of the United Kingdom. Just how much better the Swedish record is can be seen from table 4.1 and Fig 4.1 which present a form of balance sheet showing how the United Kingdom experience would have fared if it had enjoyed the mortality rates which apply in Sweden. With the exception of one age group the advantage is clearly with Sweden. From the age of one up to 44 years the differences are small, the net excess being 869 deaths in 1972. There is a large excess of infant deaths in the UK compared with Sweden, but the most striking disparity occurs from the ages of 45 to 64 years. In this age range between one-quarter and one-third of the deaths in this country in 1972 would have been avoided if the Swedish rates of mortality had applied. The way these disparities in death rates affect the expectation of life may be illustrated by considering the chances of a person aged 45 surviving a further 20 years. Whereas in Sweden 81 out of every 100 men aged 45 can expect to reach retirement age, in Scotland only 69 out of every 100 can expect to do so (table 4.1).

Some specific causes of death – international comparisons

The record of the United Kingdom as regards bronchitis mortality is a dismal one, being at present four or more times the death rates recorded in Canada, the United States, Japan, Norway and Sweden. For lung cancer Britain has the unenviable distinction of suffering the highest known death rate, both for men and for women, of any country in the world. In all developed countries heart disease is a major cause of death, particularly of men in their middle years, but here again Britain compares badly with other countries. At ages 45–64 years the death rate in Scotland is the second highest, while Northern Ireland ranks fourth and England and Wales eighth out of 27 'Western' nations.

Table 4.1 Percentage of persons aged 45 years who will NOT survive to age 65 years in Sweden and in the United Kingdom given the death rates prevailing in 1972.

Country	Males	Females
Sweden	19	11
England & Wales	27	14
Northern Ireland	29	16
Scotland	31	18

The picture is not, of course, entirely gloomy. For instance, mortality from motor vehicle accidents in Britain is roughly half the rate in Germany, though this does not imply that the number of road traffic deaths here could not be further reduced particularly among pedestrians where our record is less good. Tuberculosis, diabetes, cirrhosis of the liver and suicide are other causes of death, the rates for which are lower in Britain than in many other comparable countries. These five causes of death are, however, numerically small and in total account for only one-third of the deaths caused by lung cancer. The inference from international comparison appears inescapable: there is ample scope for improvement.

Deaths at ages 0-64 in the United Kingdom in 1972   Fig. 4·1 and number expected if the corresponding Swedish death rates had applied to the United Kingdom

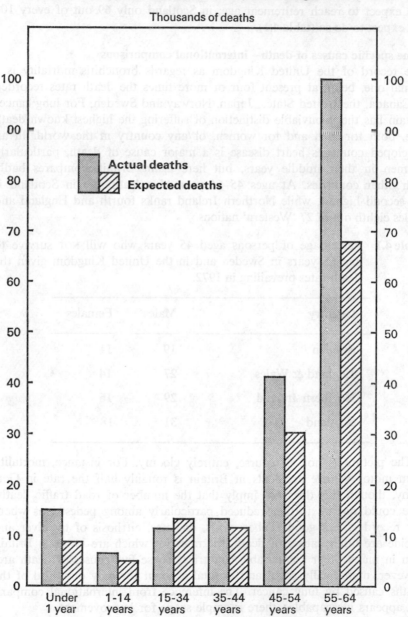

Figure 4.2

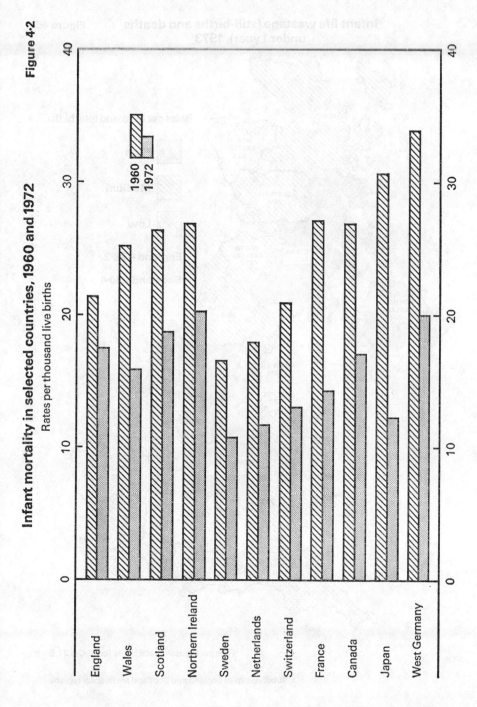

Infant mortality in selected countries, 1960 and 1972

Rates per thousand live births

Infant life wastage (still-births and deaths under 1 year), 1973

Figure 4·3

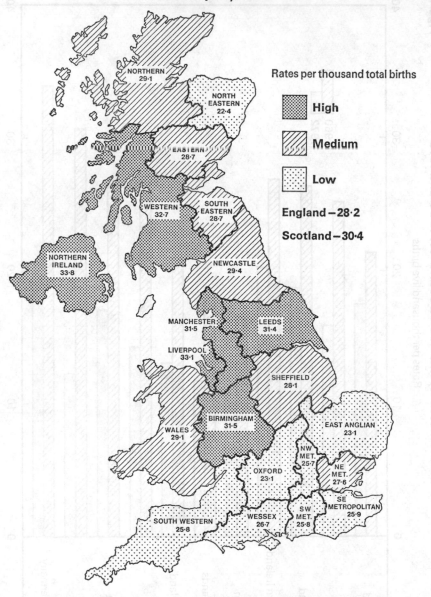

Rates per thousand total births

High

Medium

Low

England – 28·2

Scotland – 30·4

NORTHERN
29·1

NORTH
EASTERN
22·4

EASTERN
28·7

WESTERN
32·7

SOUTH
EASTERN
28·7

NORTHERN
IRELAND
33·8

NEWCASTLE
29·4

MANCHESTER
31·5

LEEDS
31·4

LIVERPOOL
33·1

SHEFFIELD
28·1

BIRMINGHAM
31·5

EAST ANGLIAN
23·1

WALES
29·1

NW
MET.
25·7

NE
MET.
27·6

OXFORD
23·1

SE
METROPOLITAN
25·9

SOUTH WESTERN
25·8

WESSEX
26·7

SW
MET.
25·8

Rate per thousand total births for GLC is 27·5

Subdivisions of England and Scotland are hospital regions

Standardised mortality ratios*, 1972
Males

Figure 4·4

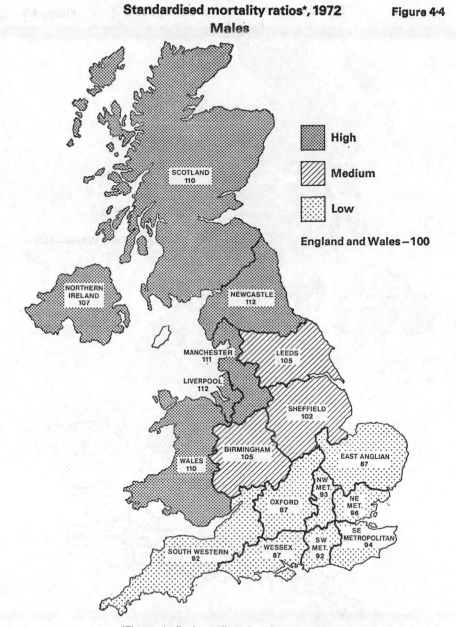

High

Medium

Low

England and Wales — 100

SCOTLAND
110

NORTHERN
IRELAND
107

NEWCASTLE
112

MANCHESTER
111

LEEDS
105

LIVERPOOL
112

SHEFFIELD
102

BIRMINGHAM
105

WALES
110

EAST ANGLIAN
87

NW
MET.
93

OXFORD
87

NE
MET.
96

SE
METROPOLITAN
94

SOUTH WESTERN
92

WESSEX
87

SW
MET.
92

*The standardised mortality ratio makes adjustment for the differences
in the age-sex composition of the population in different regions or countries.
It shows the number of deaths that occurred in the region or country
expressed as a percentage of the number that would have been expected if
the age-sex specific death rates for England and Wales as a whole had
applied to the age-sex composition of the population in the region or country.

D

Standardised mortality ratios*, 1972
Females

Figure 4·5

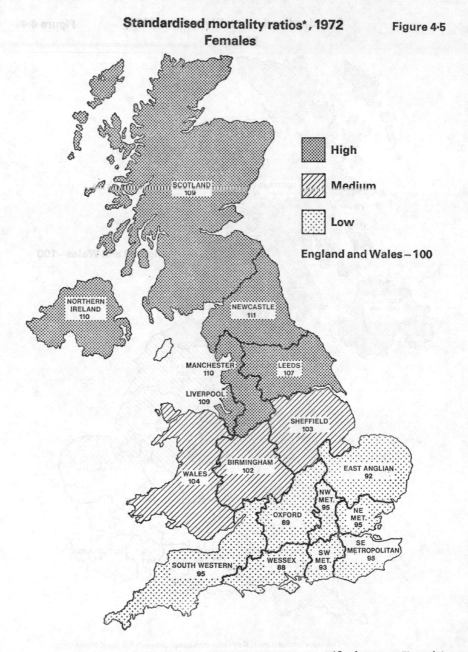

High

Medium

Low

England and Wales – 100

SCOTLAND
109

NORTHERN
IRELAND
110

NEWCASTLE
111

MANCHESTER
110

LEEDS
107

LIVERPOOL
109

SHEFFIELD
103

BIRMINGHAM
102

EAST ANGLIAN
92

WALES
104

NW
MET.
95

NE
MET.
95

OXFORD
89

SE
METROPOLITAN
95

SOUTH WESTERN
95

WESSEX
88

SW
MET.
93

*See footnote to Figure 4·4

Infant mortality – international comparisons (Fig 4.2)
Twenty years ago this country had one of the lowest rates of infant mortality but in the interim we have fallen behind other countries. Three examples will suffice; in 1960 the infant mortality rate in France was 22% above that in the United Kingdom but by 1972 the French rate was 27% below that of United Kingdom; in 1960 the rates in England and Wales and in Finland were the same, but in 1972 the Finnish rate was 34% below that in England and Wales; in 1962 the rates in Japan and Scotland were equal but 10 years later the Japan rate was nearly 40% below that of Scotland. Although infant mortality has been declining steadily in Britain over a long period the rate to-day is no better than were the rates in Scandinavia 15 years ago.

National and regional differences within the United Kingdom
The most favoured region in Britain as regards stillbirths and infant deaths in 1973 was North East Scotland and had the rates of that region applied throughout the United Kingdom there would have been in that year more than 5,000 fewer stillbirths and infant deaths (Fig 4.3). The general death rate in 1972 for males (adjusted for age) in East Anglia, Oxford and Wessex was 13% below and in Liverpool and Newcastle 12% above the England and Wales average (Fig 4.4). The disparity was not so marked for females (Fig 4.5). The mortality among males aged 55–64 in Scotland in 1972 was 17% and in Northern Ireland 10% above that in England and Wales. The death rate from lung cancer is twice as high in England and in Scotland as in Northern Ireland. Wales has the highest of the four rates for ischaemic heart disease and for bronchitis while deaths from motor accidents are relatively most frequent in Northern Ireland.

Social class differences
Mortality differentials according to socio-economic groupings have been remarked upon ever since the Registrar General first published data by social class from the census of 1911. The most recent information relates to 1961 and some of the more notable differences between the social classes at that time are set out in table 4.2. The table shows how men in the professional groups (Social Class 1) have better mortality records than almost all other groups for all diseases while labourers and unskilled workers (Social Class V) have a worse record in every category.

If the mortality to which men of working age in Social Class I were subject had applied to all men in that age range there would have been 24% or some 22,000 fewer deaths each year between 1959 and 1963.

The disparity cannot be attributed to the immediate effect of work place and work activity as such since a similar disparity exists among the wives of men in the various groups. Women aged 15–64 years whose husbands were in Social Class I were subject to a death rate (adjusted for age) 35% below the national average while women whose husbands were in unskilled occupations had a mortality 66% above the national figure.

It would be a mistake also to conclude that socio-economic gradients in mortality are solely determined by the current rate of earnings, otherwise why (1961 census) should clergymen have a lower mortality than doctors or lawyers, or agricultural labourers than merchant navy officers?

Table 4.2 Standardised mortality ratios of males aged 15–64 years for selected causes of death: England and Wales, 1961 (All classes = 100)

| | Social Class | | | | |
| | I | II | III | IV | V |
Cause of death	Profes-sional	Inter-mediate	Skilled	Partly Skilled	Unskilled
All causes	76	81	100	103	143
Tuberculosis	40	54	96	108	185
Cancer of stomach	49	63	101	114	163
Cancer of lung	53	72	107	104	148
Coronary disease	98	95	106	96	112
Bronchitis	28	50	97	116	194
Ulcer of duodenum	48	75	96	107	173
Accidents (excl. road)	43	56	87	128	193

The social class disparity in sickness records is just as striking. The volume of sickness as reported by individuals interviewed for the General Household Survey showed twice as many semi-skilled workers were on the sick list compared with employers and managers.

By industrial group the contrasts in sickness absence were even more marked, ranging from 1.6% of workers in agriculture, forestry and fishing to 11% of workers in bricks, pottery, and glass-making.

Among males aged 15 to 44 years the proportion reporting that they suffered from some form of chronic illness (not necessarily involving absence from work) was 5% among the professional classes but as high as 18% among unskilled manual workers. Men of working age in the professional classes reported losing, on average, fewer than four working days each year whereas unskilled manual workers reported losing more than eighteen days annually. If the whole of the male working population had had a sickness absence rate equivalent to that reported by the professional classes there would be an annual saving of about 100 million working days. (In 1972, a year of considerable industrial disruption, the number of working days lost because of disputes was 23.9 million). It would be a mistake in seeking to explain these disparities to ignore factors other than morbidity, for example the degree of job satisfaction that the respective groups obtain from their work and the extent to which the nature of the work prevents people with minor illnesses from staying at work. But the possibility remains of reducing the disparities by removing avoidable causes of sickness.

Environmental differences and morbidity

Many examples might be quoted to illustrate how the incidence of disease in populations varies with the environment in which they live. One of the best documented is the effect trace quantities of fluoride ion in drinking water have on the dental health of children and through much of adult life. Comparisons between communities with and without naturally occurring fluoride in the water supply have been reported from this and many other countries establishing beyond doubt the benefit to health from this environmental accident.

An example of a different kind is the direct relationship between air pollution and human disease so dramatically brought to notice in the great smog of London in 1952, when some 4,000 excess deaths occurred over about 3 weeks. Both examples also demonstrate the efficacy of deliberate intervention since the addition of fluoride to water supplies has been shown to produce the same beneficial results as where it occurs naturally, and following legislation, air pollution has virtually been eliminated in many of our populous areas. Not only will we never see a repetition of the London smog disaster but already death rates from bronchitis are on the downgrade in several of our large cities.

Table 4.3   Regional differences in the incidence of cancer of selected body-sites in Great Britain, 1963–1966.

Body site	Incidence is	
	Highest	*Lowest*
Stomach	Northern England	Wessex and Home Counties
Large bowel	Scotland	Wessex and Home Counties
Lung (females)	South-East England	Wales
Cervix	Northern England	Eastern England
Brain	Wales	Scotland
Thyroid	Scotland	North-West England
Leukaemia	South-East England	Scotland

Variations in cancer incidence

Some cancers are, of course, confined to one sex, but differences occur between the sexes in the attack rate of other forms of cancer which are common to both and these differences are strongly suggestive of differences between men and women in their exposure to carcinogens (cancer producing agents) in the environment. Cancers of the lung, larynx and urinary bladder occur several times more frequently in men, and the most acceptable explanation is the difference between the sexes in past tobacco usage. Why cancers of the stomach and rectum should be more common among men and cancers of the large bowel and thyroid gland more common among women are, on the other hand, matters for speculation.

Cancer incidence also varies between regions. There is no consistent pattern which applies to all forms of cancer (table 4.3) and with the exception of cancer of the lung, we do not know of any removable cause for these variations. Their existence however may be interpreted as evidence of potential preventability.

Variations in dental health (Table 4.4)

Dental health also provides a dramatic illustration of regional and socio-economic differences. Studies in England and Wales have shown that not only are there more people without natural teeth in the lower socio-

Table 4.4†

Total tooth loss by household social class, sex and region for people of all ages

Household Social Class	Sex	Proportion edentulous: all ages				
		The North	Wales and the South West	Midlands and East Anglia	London and the South East	England and Wales
		%	%	%	%	%
I, II and III non-manual	Male	27.4 (117)	31.9 (72)	24.3 (91)	18.5 (178)	24.0 (458)
	Female	31.5 (124)	40.3 (72)	33.3 (87)	23.9 (209)	29.9 (492)
	Both	29.5 (241)	36.1 (144)	28.7 (178)	21.4 (387)	27.1 (950)
III manual	Male	42.5 (167)	42.4 (66)	29.4 (136)	28.9 (180)	34.8 (549)
	Female	44.0 (168)	40.2 (87)	25.0 (104)	22.9 (166)	33.0 (525)
	Both	43.3 (335)	41.2 (153)	27.5 (240)	26.0 (346)	33.9 (1074)
IV non-manual, IV manual and V	Male	50.0 (100)	45.8 (48)	38.7 (80)	38.9 (95)	43.3 (323)
	Female	63.6 (118)	52.4 (42)	43.9 (82)	35.5 (107)	49.0 (349)
	Both	57.3 (218)	48.9 (90)	41.4 (162)	37.1 (202)	46.3 (672)
All* Social Classes	Male	39.3 (399)	39.4 (193)	30.2 (318)	26.7 (472)	32.9 (1382)
	Female	50.8 (465)	46.2 (238)	37.6 (311)	29.9 (536)	40.2 (1550)
	Both	45.5 (864)	43.2 (431)	33.9 (629)	28.4 (1008)	36.8 (2932)

Base numbers are given in brackets.

* These totals include the housewife, student, unemployed and unclassifiable categories which are not included elsewhere in the table.

† Reproduced from *Adult Dental Health in England and Wales in 1968* Government Social Survey HMSO.

economic groups, but that in all groups the proportion of such people increases the further you go north. The situation is generally worse among women than men in all regions and in all socio-economic groups.

No doubt a multiplicity of factors are involved in creating these discrepancies. For example, attitudes to seeking dental treatment vary from place to place and there are a higher proportion of dentists per 1,000 population in the south east than in any other region. Whatever the reason the scope for preventive action to bring all areas to the level of the best is obvious.

Hospital statistics

Morbidity in England and Wales involving hospital admission can be examined in the annual reports of the Hospital In-patient Enquiry (HIPE) and in Scotland by reference to Scottish Hospital In-Patient Statistics (SHIPS). Admission rates depend on several factors of which the volume of sickness in the population is only one. Thus, the readiness or the reluctance of people to enter hospital, the rapidity of admission and discharge, and the availability of alternative services and facilities are other important factors which influence local admission rates. It cannot therefore be deduced that a population with a high rate of hospital usage has necessarily more sickness than another population with a low rate; nor does the converse necessarily follow, that a low rate indicates a healthier population than a high rate. Nevertheless there are striking differences between regions of the country to be seen in the HIPE reports. In 1972 the region with the largest number of hospital beds in daily occupation in relation to the size of its population had a ratio 25% above, and the region with the lowest number a ratio of 13% below the national average. Were there too many beds in the one region or too few in the other? Or were the numbers about right given the prevalence of disease in the two regions? If that was the case why did the prevalence differ so much?

The disparity in fact is substantial. If the whole country needs hospital provision on the scale of the region with the highest ratio an extra 45,000 beds are required; but if the ratio in the lowest region were both adequate and attainable nationally some 23,500 beds are redundant. Unfortunately we do not know to what extent these extremes reflect preventable illness. For the reasons stated we cannot interpret differences in admission rates as simply due to differences in the volume of disease let alone disease which we know how to prevent. By the same token we cannot be certain that the regional disparities that undoubtedly exist do not arise in part from preventable disease.

Some general thoughts
This chapter is intended to set the reader asking why these differences between nations, within countries, between social and occupational groups and between hospital regions should exist. It is obviously not possible in this brief survey to do more than indicate the complexities of the subject but a birds eye view may be of interest. The following is a list of some of the more important factors.

a Genetic factors
b Climatic factors
c Environmental factors in the general environment
d Environmental factors in the occupational environment
e Life-style (for example diet, exercise, use of alcohol and tobacco)
f Quality, quantity and cost to the individual of health and social services provided
g The use made of services
h Educational factors
i Economic factors

The importance of each factor varies with the problem. Chapters I and II demonstrated that such factors as improvements in the environment (housing and sanitation) and in nutrition probably played a major part in reducing mortality from some of the infectious diseases of childhood and from tuberculosis, cholera and typhoid. Other factors enumerated above may well have been of less importance.

To turn to an existing problem, when considering infant mortality the whole complex of medical and social factors come into play. Why has the position of Sweden been consistently so much better than our own? And why has the infant mortality rate been lower within the United Kingdom in social class I than in social class V; and why, despite all the changes in the past fifty years, does the disparity remain – at least in Scotland (we have no recent data for the rest of the United Kingdom) – as wide as ever? Socio-economic factors seem to be of great importance here, but how do they act? Housing, nutrition, life-style, education and income may all play a part. It is said that the organisation of society in such countries as Sweden reduces the social class differences. This may well be so, but it is noteworthy that other nations with widely differing structures of society have caught up and passed us in the past few years. Perhaps one of the more important factors is use of services, and it certainly seems to be true that the lower socio-economic group mothers make less use of the preventive health services both before and after delivery. This in turn may be connected with education.

If other examples were discussed in detail the further speculation would be as fascinating as it would be time consuming. The general point that seems to emerge, however, is that with the current problems facing us there are no general sets of answers such as the sanitary revolution and the control of infectious diseases provided for our 19th century ancestors. In some cases our present problems of prevention seem to call for more research into causation. In many the major issue is the amount of resources needed to carry out a programme and the question of which projects deserve to be given preference in using the limited amounts of money and equally important skilled manpower available locally for preventive work. In yet other cases the key factor may be the need to educate the individual so that he can help himself. And all too often two or more of these factors are combined. The following chapters therefore seek to look at the practicalities of prevention in this era and the factors which often make it difficult, in particular subjects, to make the progress which at first sight seems obviously necessary and possible.

CHAPTER V Practicalities of prevention

Introduction

It is one thing to identify the causes of disease and quite another to decide whether, and if so how, to remove and modify those causes. Serious questions arise as to whether legislation is justified or whether to concentrate on health education as the most appropriate approach. There are areas where preventive action may be considered by some an unjustified intrusion into individual freedom; it is not always possible to be sure that a certain course of action will prove to be beneficial, yet failure to act may be even more damaging; and occasionally traditional safeguards lose their relevance. These are the kind of issues of special concern at present and we shall consider some of them in this chapter by reference to a number of specific topics.

Smoking diseases

No one can seriously doubt any longer that the habit of cigarette smoking has been directly responsible for an enormous amount of preventable disease and untimely death in this country. There are, however, a few hopeful signs. As already stated in Chapter III, fewer men smoke than hitherto; since 1960 there has been a big switch away from plain to filter cigarettes; the tar yield of the average cigarette is lower; the death rate from lung cancer among males in the younger age groups has ceased to rise; and cigarette smoking is becoming less common in social classes I and II. But there are ominous signs too. More women have taken up smoking and this trend can only give rise to concern. Smoking during pregnancy damages the chances of healthy development of the unborn child, and one estimate suggested that over a thousand foetal and infant deaths in Britain in 1970 were associated with smoking in pregnancy.

Of course preventive medicine has encountered difficulties almost as large in the past. The Victorian sanitary reformers faced resistance to the introduction of legislation aimed at improving the sewage system but much of the opposition they encountered came from people who did not understand the dangers of the existing situation. The same is not true of smoking and this underlines the central dilemma facing those who wish to reduce the risks to health from such a dangerous habit. Today most smokers continue to smoke cigarettes fully aware that they run a risk of killing themselves, slowly and probably painfully. Much money has been spent on anti-smoking propaganda, though it is a trifle by comparison with that spent by the tobacco companies on promoting sales, and young people continue to take up the habit, discounting the risks or possibly believing that they will be able to give it up before ill-health strikes.

Despite the publicity given to the hazards of cigarette smoking and the attempts made to assist smokers to stop, it is very difficult to get people to change their smoking habits once these have become ingrained. Without relaxing our efforts at health education we must therefore consider the adoption of other lines of attack if we are serious about preventing smoking-related disease.

The development of what are hoped to be less dangerous cigarettes is one approach being pursued in this country and elsewhere. Filter cigarettes have already reduced average tar and nicotine yields and, while tobacco substitutes may give rise to further reductions (and thus it is postulated to a lower risk of disease), it remains to be seen whether cigarettes containing these materials will be any less damaging than the conventional cigarette.

Recent opinion polls suggest that a majority of people in this country are in favour of some form of stricter controls over cigarettes; though they differ as to the form that increased control should take. At present the tobacco trade is subject in several countries to more stringent oversight than in Britain. In Norway, for example, a Tobacco Act has just come into force which imposes a complete ban on advertising of tobacco products in all media, including the use of tobacco in connection with the advertising of other goods and services; an obligation for cigarette packets to carry a more strongly worded warning than is in use in Britain; and which confers on the Minister of Social Affairs powers to regulate the content, weight, filters and packaging of tobacco products. A number of other countries also have legislation regulating the advertising, sale and packaging of cigarettes. In some countries smoking is prohibited by law in schools and hospitals in recognition of the singular responsibility of the teaching and the health professions not to encourage the habit by their own example.

One important point to make is that a reduction in cigarette smoking would be reflected within a relatively short time – certainly within 10 years – in a reduction in smoking-related diseases, particularly coronary disease, as has already been demonstrated from analysis of the mortality experience of British doctors.

The Government has said that in its view what is needed is machinery analagous to that provided for in the Medicines Act. This would enable action regulating such matters as the yield of tar and other noxious substances, health warnings on advertisements and packets, restriction of promotion of sales, and the use of substitutes and additives, to be based on advice from an expert and independent advisory committee after consultation with interests likely to be substantially affected.

Coronary heart disease

Coronary (or ischaemic) heart disease is the foremost cause of death of middle-aged males in Great Britain; 43 per cent of all male deaths between the ages of 45 and 64 years are due to this one cause. Many of these deaths occur suddenly and unexpectedly but ischaemic heart disease is also the cause of much hospital treatment. About 3,500 hospital beds are in use every day in Great Britain for the treatment of patients under the age of 65 with this condition. Up to that age men patients outnumber women by three to one, just as male death rates exceed those of females.

Despite the immense volume of research into the causes of coronary disease, a measure of uncertainty remains about the underlying pathology and there is a lack of agreement on the degree of effectiveness of preventive measures. It is acknowledged that certain characteristics are risk factors in the sense that individuals possessing them are more likely to suffer a coronary attack than are individuals who do not. It does not necessarily follow, however, that if the individuals possessing the characteristic were somehow to lose it, their risk of attack would come to approximate that of persons who had never possessed the characteristic in the first place. With respect to one risk factor only could it be said with certainty that removing it reduces the risk substantially: there is good evidence from several studies that cigarette smokers who give up the habit will subsequently run a lower risk of heart attacks. The other main risk factors are obesity, lack of exercise, high blood pressure, high blood fat levels, and a family history of heart trouble. None of us can do much about the last of these but, regarding the others, three observations may be made.

First, the risk factors are themselves highly associated one with another. For example, obese people usually take little exercise, and so on.

Second, statistical associations tell us little about the size of the risk for any given individual. Many people with more than one of these undesirable attributes never suffer heart attacks, at least up to an advanced age, while some people displaying none of these characteristics are struck down while still comparatively young.

Third, we have little real evidence as yet to show that getting rid of these attributes reduces the statistical risk. Some trials on these lines have been conducted – others are in progress – but the results have not been entirely convincing. While therefore it would seem sound common sense to take preventive action with regard to these risk factors, the evidence we have falls short of proof that the desired result will follow. In a word, there are plausible but not proven means of reducing morbidity and mortality from heart disease in middle life.

'People who are naturally very fat', observed Hippocrates 2,400 years ago, 'are apt to die earlier than those who are slender', and modern actuarial statistics support that view and the life assurance houses act accordingly. Similarly men who take regular and vigorous exercise usually enjoy better health, and have on average lower blood pressures and lower blood cholesterol levels than men who do not. Even allowing for any bias due to self-selection (giving rise to the objection that the correct deduction is that the healthy take strenuous exercise rather than it is strenuous exercise that makes them healthy) there is an inherent plausibility in the argument, sufficient to convince many people that sloth and gluttony are still deadly sins, and to mend their ways accordingly.

The role of diet in causing coronary disease seems to be particularly contentious. There is agreement among the experts that there might well be advantages if people were to reduce their consumption of animal fat and of sugar, but expert opinion is divided, for example, on whether to recommend greater use of polyunsaturated fats in order to prevent coronary attacks.

There are those, indeed, who with great daring ask the question whether we really should try to prevent coronary heart disease? They suggest that the most we should aim for is to delay the initial attack, or if it should have come at a relatively early age and the patient survives, to delay a recurrence. To judge by recent mortality data (Table 5.1) this is what appears to be happening in Sweden, for it is only at advanced ages that the death rate of males in Sweden from this cause exceeds that in the United Kingdom.

In summary, there are several forms of behaviour which are associated with lower than average risk of coronary disease. Probably the most important single factor which men from their youth onwards should ponder is cigarette smoking, with exercise and obesity next in order of importance. To the extent therefore that coronary heart disease is determined by a man's life style the prime responsibility for his own health falls on the individual. The role of the health professions and of government is limited to ensuring that the public have access to such knowledge as is available about the importance of personal habit on health and that at the very least no obstacles are placed in the way of those who decide to act on that knowledge.

Table 5.1 Death rates of males per 100,000 population from ischaemic heart disease at ages 35 years and upwards, in England, Wales, Scotland, Northern Ireland and Sweden, in 1972.

Age group	England	Wales	Scotland	N. Ireland	Sweden
35–44	65	89	95	70	25
45–54	286	360	360	369	152
55–64	728	891	963	940	528
65–74	1,694	1,991	2,049	1,942	1,564
75 & over	3,628	4,330	4,452	4,186	4,755

A possible direct involvement of government can be foreseen only in one direction. It has been found that people living in hard water areas tend to have less heart disease than those in soft water areas. When the relationship between hard and soft water and heart disease is clarified it may turn out that some constituent is specifically harmful, in which case it should be removed if present; or specifically beneficial, when it could be added if absent from a public water supply. That point has not yet been reached and the only valid advice that can be offered at present is that the responsible authorities should think very carefully before deciding to reduce the hardness of a water supply.

Fluoridation and dental decay
Very few preventive measures are as effective or are so easy to implement as the fluoridation of water supplies. The addition (where it does not occur naturally) of minute traces of fluoride to drinking water has been established beyond doubt as being completely safe and the most effective method of substantially reducing the incidence of dental caries in the community. This has received further authoritative endorsement in the report 'Fluoride, Teeth and Health' published by the Royal College of Physicians in January 1976.

Yet of all recent initiatives in preventive medicine this has been in

Britain, though not in other countries (eg the United States, Canada, the Republic of Ireland) the most disappointing. Throughout the United Kingdom only 8.6 per cent of the population is now receiving water supplies containing fluoride (in those areas where it does not occur naturally). To give the greatest protection fluoridated water must be consumed by children and young people from birth throughout the period of tooth development. All the evidence from overseas countries where fluoride has been present in water supplies for long periods indicates that benefits persist throughout life especially if complemented by sound habits of diet and oral hygiene.

The safety of the procedure has been amply demonstrated by the health records of many communities that have for a long time used water supplies containing fluoride, often in excess of the optimal level for the prevention of dental disease.

Convincing evidence of the efficacy of fluoride in reducing dental decay can be seen in those areas where enlightened authorities have gone ahead with fluoridation. Eleven years after its introduction in study areas in this country, it was shown that among children aged 8, 9 and 10, 34% were completely free of dental decay compared with only 15% before fluoride was added. The amount of decay in milk teeth of children aged 3 to 7 inclusive fell by as much as a half. The changes are in marked contrast to the dental health of children in 'control' areas where fluoride was not added. Here decay fell by only one fifth in the 3 to 7 age group and only one twentieth in the group aged 8 to 10. This slower trend towards better dental health even without fluoride can be attributed to better dental care during the same period.

Of course fluoride can be administered on an individual basis by the use of tablets, and better dental health could be assured if only parents discouraged children from eating sweets, lollipops, drinks containing sugar and so on. For practical purposes neither is acceptable. Experience has shown that the necessary degree of persistence and supervision in giving their children tablets, is achieved only by a minority of parents and a childhood without sweets may well be regarded by many as a fate worse than an adulthood without teeth.

Certainly it is advisable to maintain teeth in good condition by regular brushing and avoiding sweet things between meals but sound habits of hygiene and diet can be successful only if applied to teeth which are basically strong and healthy, and these measures and water fluoridation should not be regarded as substitutes one for the other, but rather as complementary.

The cost benefit issue in relation to fluoridation is considered in Chapter VII, Page 85.

Road traffic accidents

About 7,200 people are killed and some 85,000 seriously injured on roads in the United Kingdom each year. In 1971 the number of road casualties admitted to hospital in England, Scotland and Wales was over 100,000. Not all these injuries proved to be serious, but even so more than 3,000 hospital beds were in constant use for their treatment. It was estimated that the total cost to the country – hospital treatment being but a part – of all road traffic accidents including those not involving serious injury in that year was close to £500 millions. (See page 85). Young people aged 15 to 24 years are at the greatest risk and given the prevailing traffic accident rates in this age range, one out of every 50 school leavers will be killed on the roads or seriously injured and perhaps maimed for life before he is 10 years older.

Two measures of proven effectiveness in reducing this toll of death and injury are the use of seat belts and a further tightening of the law relating to driving and drinking.

The wearing of seat belts is now compulsory in several countries (Australia, Belgium, France, Luxembourg, the Netherlands, New Zealand, Spain, Sweden and USSR) and is shortly to be introduced in others (West Germany, Switzerland). The benefits if Britain were to follow suit would be immediate and substantial. Using data for 1971 it can be estimated that about 14,000 fatal and serious injuries would be averted each year if all drivers and front seat passengers used seat belts at all times.

The difficulty here, of course, is that some people do not like wearing seat belts and that to force them to do so would be an infringement of personal liberty. Failure to wear a seat belt does not, after all, pose a threat to others, though avoidable injury imposes an unnecessary burden on the health services. The argument is not dissimilar to that over the enforced wearing of crash helmets for motor-cyclists, but legislation for that purpose was enacted all the same.

The introduction of the breath test, and the prescribed limit offence, in 1967 was widely accepted, probably in view of the serious threat posed by the drunken driver to other road users. It resulted immediately in a remarkable fall in the number of serious accidents and, in the period since, it has been claimed that 200,000 casualties, including 5,000 deaths, have been avoided as a direct result of the Road Safety Act 1967.

Unfortunately it is evident that the law is not as effective as it was. The proportion of casualties that occur late at night ('the drinking hours') has been rising and is now about the level it was before the Act came into force. Prior to 1967 the proportion of drivers killed with blood alcohol levels above the legal limit of 80 mg per ml was 25 per cent.

E

Immediately following the introduction of the breath tests the proportion fell to 15 per cent: it has now risen to 34 per cent. The proportion represents about 900 dead drivers each year. In addition, account has to be taken of the drivers with illegal blood alcohol levels who were seriously injured and occupants of cars or other road users killed or injured, in order to arrive at some estimate of the cost of drunken driving.

The number of convictions has risen every year since the Act, but the deterrent effect has clearly been lost. One answer would be to devote more effort to enforcement, which might be rendered easier if the restrictions on the police power to test were removed. Another is to pay more attention to alcoholics and 'problem drinkers', whom some now believe to form a large proportion of drinking drivers: at present the consequences of conviction are not sufficient to break their habit. Finally, further publicity and education are needed on an issue where public apathy is still very great.

The dilemmas of uncertainty

Just as life, according to Samuel Butler, is the art of drawing sufficient conclusions from insufficient premises so also many decisions with implications for disease prevention have to be taken despite a measure of uncertainty about the consequences. The recurring dilemma is whether or not to act on the basis of inadequate information. Some would say that the 'coronary' story outlined above points up this dilemma. But the difficulty can be even more acute in attempting to assess the evidence for a potential chemical or physical hazard either in the environment generally or in an industrial setting both because of the complexity of issues which could be involved and because the banning of a material will deprive the community of a product which is being found useful, in one way or another. It is often a matter of balancing a possible risk against a known advantage.

As regards numbers, many tens of thousands of new chemicals or new formulations of old ones are proposed to be introduced into the environment somewhere in the world every year. If only a very small proportion are suspected of presenting a possible threat to health many evaluations, often calling for judgements of great difficulty, would still have to be made annually.

A recent example was a report that certain hair dyes might give rise to cancer. The chemicals in question had in fact been shown to be capable of inducing cell changes in certain bacteria. But testing-techniques of this kind using bacterial systems or cell culture methods are relatively new and, more important, are somewhat remote from the human condition so that a positive result in a bacterial system cannot be taken as implying that there is necessarily a risk to man. It is therefore at least arguable whether one should, on the basis of such evidence, deprive society of the use of such products.

Another example of the dilemma arises from the use of nitrites as preservatives in canned meat. This is a practice which has been widely followed for many years, among other reasons because nitrites prevent bacterial growth, especially that which could lead to botulism, a deadly form of food poisoning.

Under certain circumstances nitrites can combine with certain naturally occurring substances to form compounds known as nitrosamines which, in animal experiments, have been found to be potent cancer-producing substances. There is no evidence that nitrosamines can induce cancer in man and this is not surprising since only a score of substances are definitely known to give rise to human cancer, compared with a thousand or more compounds of proven carcinogenicity in one animal species or another. Clearly it is necessary for the Government to ensure that research continues in order to gain as much knowledge as possible about the real risk, to take advice from its own scientists and from panels of advisers who will assess the benefits of use in relation to hazards, and to maintain a close and continuing watch on the situation. Do we, in the meantime, discontinue the use of a substance of proven value against food poisoning because of a possible, and on present evidence remote, risk of another hazard?

Another difficulty that recurs is the question of safe levels. For example, a few cases of a rare form of liver cancer have recently been traced to industrial exposure to the chemical vinyl chloride monomer used in the manufacture of PVC, a plastic in common use, among other purposes, for the packaging of food in order to keep it hygienic and free from infection. It is therefore necessary to decide, first, what level of exposure to the monomer should be permitted in the manufacturing process, balancing the gravity of the risk against the small numbers likely to incur it and the fact that to set too low a level could render production impossible. The second issue is what trace level of monomer should be permitted in the finished product if used to wrap food, bearing in mind that too low a level might rule out the use of PVC altogether for this purpose. In this instance it so happens that with the full co-operation of the chemical industry the residual levels of monomer in PVC packaging have been reduced to barely detectable levels and to this extent the area of uncertainty has been reduced. But the general problem remains; in many cases the Government, and society as a whole, must, on the basis of the best knowledge available at the time weigh a known benefit against a potential disadvantage which may be very remote but could be serious if it arose.

The dilemmas of uncertainty are by no means peculiar to chemical and physical hazards. For example, there is no conclusive scientific evidence one way or the other about the effect on the mental health of children of violence in television. What should parents do? Today's problems are sometimes the consequence of yesterday's policies (there are very few advocates of high rise housing around any more) and the best we can do is to ensure that today's policies are based on today's knowledge. In the long run the acid test of the correct course, whether in the rearing of children or the use of new chemicals, is what happens to the individuals concerned. In addition to specific research we must be prepared to take full advantage of the casual human 'experiments' that are in progress all the time.

Mind and body

The first part of this chapter had been concerned with the physical environment and its physical effects (eg road-accidents, fluoride in water) as well as with physical ailments such as coronary thrombosis, chronic bronchitis or cancer of the lung. Of course anyone who has ever been seriously ill or injured is aware that even in such acute conditions the effects on the mind are profound and if we separate mind and body it is only for convenience. Just as we cannot really separate mind and body so we cannot separate man from the society he lives in. This chapter will conclude with a brief look at three problems which can be gathered together under the heading of mental ill-health but it must be stressed that this is purely a convenience and the discussion will make clear the interaction of mind, body and society.

ALCOHOLISM

The level of alcoholism and other drink-related problems in any given society appears to be closely linked with the level of overall consumption and may therefore be affected by the controls over the use of alcohol exerted by that society, whether legal, fiscal or social. Legal controls are concerned with such matters as the production and sale of alcohol and conditions of sale (licensing, opening hours, age of starting to drink legally in public). Fiscal controls rest on the theory that total consumption of alcohol rises when the price, in real terms, falls and vice versa and that the incidence of alcoholism is directly correlated with consumption. Social controls are the result of attitudes to alcohol and its consumption and may well be the most important of the three.

The attitudes of a society towards alcohol may be reflected in its legal and fiscal controls, whose nature and strength may in turn influence, reinforce or weaken that society's social controls. The best combination of strategies for our society, and the attitudes to alcohol which should be encouraged in it, are matters which deserve public discussion. The role of advertising in helping to form our attitudes to alcohol is among the matters to be debated: voluntary codes relating to drink advertisements already exist but there is as yet little experience of their working. Health education designed to strengthen social controls is, however, a long term and important task.

In addition to these long-term strategies, there remains the short-term need to help the problem drinker. Public attitudes play a crucial part in this. There is need for a general awareness of the nature of alcoholism and of the available sources of help, so that those with drinking problems and their families are encouraged to seek assistance at an early stage.

MENTAL HANDICAP

In most cases of mental handicap the cause is not known. Severe handicap occurs in about 4 per 1,000 live births and in only a minority of cases are there demonstrable inherited or environmental factors. Among this minority are Down's Syndrome (mongolism) which accounts for about one-third of all cases of severe mental handicap. The number of mongol births has been declining and the potential for further reduction is examined in Chapter VI. An increasing number of rare biochemical defects with a genetic basis are being recognised; screening of the newborn for phenylketonuria, the commonest of these rare defects is now standard practice (see Chapter VI).

Environmental factors include german measles and certain other infections in the mother and exposure to X-rays of the unborn child. Childbirth and the period immediately thereafter may in some cases involve risk of brain damage. Haemolytic disease of the newborn can cause mental defects and the successful efforts to reduce its incidence were discussed in Chapter II.

In early infancy and childhood infections such as meningitis and encephalitis and non-accidental injury ('baby-battering') may sometimes result in severe mental handicap.

It is therefore possible by specific preventive measures to reduce the incidence of severe mental handicap. Vaccination against measles and rubella, genetic counselling, family planning, skilled midwifery and special care of the newborn are practical ways of achieving this end. In addition to the recognised health and social services the importance of special attention to high-risk families should be stressed.

Estimates of incidence of mild degrees of mental handicap vary, but all are agreed that it is much more frequent than severe handicap. There is clear evidence that the overall performance of a child with mild mental retardation can be depressed by poor social conditions and educational opportunities. Where, in addition, there are other defects perhaps of vision or hearing, the full potential of the child may be significantly and permanently reduced. Improved housing, wider educational and vocational opportunities, good medical and social services, and effective early detection and assessment services could all contribute to ameliorate the effects of mild mental handicap.

DEPRESSION

Mental illness is, in this country today, a problem of major importance. In England alone every year some 5 million people consult their general practitioner about a mental health problem and 600,000 receive specialist psychiatric services; for its treatment 110,000 hospital beds are in use and it is responsible for the loss of 24 million working days. But the application of the principles of prevention in the field of mental hygiene is hampered by difficulties of definition, by the confusion that exists between deviant or disturbed behaviour on the one hand and abnormal mental functioning on the other. There is also a lack of precise knowledge of causation which means that prevention can be discussed only in broad general terms. To some mental health means no more than the absence of obvious insanity, to others it means the condition enjoyed by the well adjusted person who is functioning effectively as a member of society. A wide range of social and environmental circumstances may be associated with an increased vulnerability to mental illness and the precise weight to be attached to them can rarely be established. It would be wrong to pretend that we are anywhere near being able to draw up a positive plan for a society that would be conducive to mental health.

This document is not the place to attempt any wide-ranging review of this difficult field but it may be useful for the purposes of illustration to refer to a specific and all too common manifestation of mental ill-health, depression. Depression may range from normal sadness through deep gloom with suicidal intent to the extremes of mute withdrawal and, given the 'declension' as Shakespeare has called it from sadness to madness, it is not always easy to distinguish between what may be a normal if severe reaction to adversity and what may be a pathological degree of distress. In practice depressive illness is often preceded by some event involving a deep sense of loss. The death of a spouse, the break-up of a marriage, the damage to self-confidence that a disabling illness or mutilating accident can occasion, are frequent fore-runners of depression. These are the tribulations that await many on life's way and as such they must sometimes be accepted as unavoidable; the most we can do in such events is to help people to meet them and in particular to recognise when an individual appears to be at risk of actual mental illness as a consequence. There may be scope for counselling services to help with family problems, to prepare for redundancy or retirement, to support the bereaved, and to encourage the rehabilitation of the sick or injured.

Depression is also found to occur more frequently at certain times in people's lives. Thus, adolescence may bring violent swings in mood which make for a stormy period of development of the personality; and it is in an attempt to cope with such problems that youth advisory services have been set up in some areas. Childbirth and the period immediately after is another period when depressive illness can develop and this places a particular responsibility on those undertaking ante-natal and post-natal care to recognise the onset of trouble so as to give the patient the benefit of early treatment. In middle life women at the menopause are not infrequently subject to depression which may call for special forms of treatment; and finally, depression is all too often seen in the elderly especially those living alone.

Suicide and attempted suicide are often the result of depression. Many contemplate suicide and about 4,000 suicides were recorded in Britain in 1972. One method that has been devised to try and help those in dire distress is the 'crisis centre' while voluntary bodies like the Samaritans offer in many areas a 24 hour service to people in need of support.

Active treatment of depression is in itself a form of prevention to the extent that it prevents the patient's condition from deteriorating and assists a return to normal functioning. Nowhere is this aspect more important perhaps that in the cases of depression associated with childbirth since these distressing cases so often have long-lasting and damaging effects on the family as a whole.

Brief though it has been this resumé of some of the features of depressive illness should serve to indicate how, despite the complexities of the field, it is still possible to recognise that some people are more at risk than others, that the onset of mental illness can sometimes be anticipated, and that those affected can often be helped. But it must be admitted that our over-riding need at this time is for a more profound understanding of the intricate interactions between the individual, his inheritance and his upbringing and the environment, social and physical in which he lives. For it is when these interactions go awry that mental ill-health results.

CHAPTER VI

Looking for trouble

Diagnosis and detection

Screening, the deliberate examination of substantial segments of the population – even the entire population – in a search for disease at its earliest stages is a logical extension of the role of preventive medicine and one which is, rightly or wrongly, becoming increasingly in vogue.

So far this document has been concerned mostly with the role of primary prevention, that is anticipating where disease might strike and taking steps to ensure that, as far as possible, it cannot or that if it does its effects will be minimal. The essence of secondary prevention is to go out and look for disease at a stage when the victim may not be aware that he has it or even that he is liable to get it.[1]

Of course there are occasions when these two purposes of preventive medicine coincide, as for example when contacts are traced and examined in the control of tuberculosis or venereal disease so that by treating the infecting individual, the further spread of infection from that source can be prevented. For the most part, however, secondary prevention is the search for disease in a person who appears to be perfectly healthy.

The view is widely held today that early diagnosis of disease once we are aware something is wrong is beneficial because it makes it possible to start treatment before the disease process has progressed to the stage of being irreversible – in other words while the disease is yet curable. This is why we are often urged not to delay in seeking advice when we notice something amiss.

Equally it is logical, particularly when dealing with chronic and de-

[1] For the sake of completeness mention might be made here of tertiary prevention. This is concerned with minimising the disability arising out of existing disease or injury. Thus, the continuing treatment of established disease to arrest its progress is a form of tertiary prevention. So too are those methods of treatment aimed at the rehabilitation of the patient who has recovered from an acute attack of disease or in whose case the disease process has been wholly or partially arrested.

generative diseases, to deduce that if, at a given point in the course of its development, a disease declares itself by causing symptoms it must already have been present for some time beforehand and that, given a sensitive enough test, the disease might have been detected even in this pre-symptomatic phase. If early diagnosis when we notice something amiss is a good thing, the argument goes, then early detection before we notice something is amiss must be even better.

There is a distinction to be drawn between screening and diagnosis. A positive result in a screening test does not establish a diagnosis – but it does raise the presumption that disease is present which must be confirmed or refuted by further investigation as a prelude to treatment if need be.

The importance of the distinction between diagnosis and screening lies in the relationship between the screener and the screened. Whereas early diagnosis depends on the patient seeking advice, in a screening programme the promoters take the initiative and adopt what has been aptly described as an 'evangelical' position (Matthew, 22: 9,10[1]). In so doing they assume responsibilities of a different order from those of the physician whose help a patient has sought.

It can be argued, therefore, that population screening is justified only when a benefit can be conferred on those responding to the invitation to come forward to be screened. (There may be an exception to this rule where the public interest is involved as, for example, when waterworks employees are screened to detect typhoid carriers). In general, most people would agree that to offer screening for a disease for which no treatment exists would be unethical. Equally, if the only treatment available is for the relief of symptoms there is no advantage to the affected individual in detecting his disease before symptoms have appeared. Even where an accepted method of treatment exists for the disease in question, the advocate of screening must be prepared to show that starting treatment at the presymptomatic stage will modify the natural course of the disease in the patient's favour to a greater extent than treatment instituted only after symptoms have appeared.

Unfortunately screening has appealed to some in recent years as a panacea offering advantages far in excess of those which can be justly claimed for it. But there are problems which should not be underestimated. The sheer scale and cost of endeavouring to provide regular

[1] ' "Go out to the main thoroughfares, and invite everyone you can find to the wedding". The servants went out into the streets, and collected all they could find, good and bad alike. So the hall was packed with guests'. (New English Bible, second edition © 1970 by permission of Oxford & Cambridge University Presses.)

screenings for all diseases for the whole population are sufficient to make it utterly impractical, quite apart from any considerations of how effective it might or might not be. And there are other limiting factors.

It is, for example often taken for granted that the limits of 'normality' are well defined but this is not necessarily so, particularly when dealing with a variable such as blood pressure where the range of normality is wide. There are indeed some experts who would challenge the whole concept of 'normal'; and it is certainly true that the earlier in the progression from normal to abnormal that one seeks for the first signs of abnormality, the more uncertain the boundary and the more difficult the task.

Again there are few screening tests which produce results which are consistently reliable. In any group of people subjected to a screening examination there will be those who give a positive result and in whom disease is confirmed on subsequent examination. They are known as 'true positives'. However there will be others who will give a positive result on screening but who will subsequently prove on investigation to be free from disease. They are 'false positives'.

In exactly the same way there will be uncertainties in the initial results of those in whom screening is negative. Some (the 'true negatives') will in fact have no disease but others ('the false negatives') will prove to have the disease despite being reassured by the screening test.

The very nature of early detection techniques probably makes such outcomes inevitable without necessarily invalidating the procedures, but the potential for wasted effort is immediately apparent and underlines the need for screening to be concentrated on groups of the population in whom specific diseases might be expected.

High risk groups
Obviously only half the population need be considered as potential subjects for cervical cytology (the 'smear' test for pre-cancer of neck of womb). But even among females the very young and those who have had a hysterectomy (removal of the womb) can be excluded, as not being at risk. The process of selection can be carried further since it is known that the probability of cervical cancer among women who have never been sexually active is negligible. The more precisely one can concentrate on that sub-group within the general population that is at highest risk, the more efficient the screening programme will be. And the more expensive and onerous the screening procedure with its attendant diagnostic follow-up, the more worthwhile does selective screening become.

There are clearly two requirements. First, it must be possible to identify the high risk individual by virtue of some characteristic (sex, age, occupation etc) that has been shown by epidemiological studies to be statistically associated with an enhanced probability of developing the disease; and second, the individuals so identified must be persuaded to come forward for screening. In practice it is often easier to meet the first requirement than the second.

For reasons we do not completely understand some people are distinctly reluctant to come forward for screening even if they belong in a high risk group and research to seek ways of overcoming their fears is in progress.

Acceptability

A test, if it is to be applied on a population scale, should be acceptable to the public. Thus, it should be free of risk, or if not, the risk involved in being tested should be small compared with the risk of not being tested. The test should not cause undue inconvenience or distress as otherwise the public will not respond. For large scale application the cost of the test must be reasonable in relation to the benefits to be expected from screening. For example, the large bowel and the rectum are among the parts of the body frequently affected by cancer and three-quarters of all cancers of these sites are accessible to direct examination by a technique known as sigmoidoscopy which can be used for screening. It should be possible therefore to detect many of these cancers at a presymptomatic stage provided persons aged, say, 50 years and upwards (ie the age at which these particular cancers start to become relatively prevalent) submit at intervals to sigmoidoscopy.

However sigmoidoscopy involves the insertion of a tube into the anus and inside the intestine for a distance of several inches. It is doubtful if the public could ever be persuaded to accept such a programme, which is perhaps as well since the resources and expert manpower required are such that population screening by sigmoidoscopy is never likely to be feasible. It so happens that there is in any case no evidence that the presymptomatic detection of cancer of the bowel or rectum would improve the chances of cure or the quality of life after treatment. It might achieve either or both of these desirable objectives – or it might achieve neither.

Effectiveness

To launch a programme of population screening without adequate grounds for believing it to be effective could be an irresponsible diversion of scarce resources which might have been deployed to better purpose in some other direction. Evidence of effectiveness is best provided by a controlled trial in which the experience of a screened group is compared with that of a group otherwise comparable which is not screened. Depending on the disease in question such a trial may have to be conducted on a large scale and for a long time, yet few screening procedures have been properly tested in this way.

Cervical cytology (examination of samples of cells taken from the neck of the womb) for example, was introduced after much research in this and in other countries in response to intense public pressure, but before its effectiveness had been fully demonstrated. The test has however identified abnormalities, many of which were probably pre-cancerous, in thousands of women who were subsequently treated and a proportion of them were saved from developing cancer. Coincidentally the incidence of cervical cancer has diminished in recent years for reasons which (as suggested earlier) are at present obscure, so it is difficult to be sure to what extent the screening programme itself has saved lives. It remains nevertheless a safeguard and reassurance for those women who take advantage of the simple procedure.

Frequency of screening

For some purposes an individual needs to be screened only once – screening newborn infants for phenylketonuria is an example – but other screening programmes require the tests to be repeated since the fact that a person is free of disease on one occasion is no guarantee he or she may not develop the disease at some future time. The length of the interval between tests should ideally be dictated by the rate of progression from normality to detectable abnormality. This rate is, however, likely to vary between individuals and an ideal screening programme would take account of this variation. In practice the interval chosen will depend more on the resources that can be devoted to the programme, on the public response to repeated testing, and on administrative feasibility rather than on theoretical considerations.

The earliest attempt in this country at mass medical examination of a whole segment of the population was inaugurated as long ago as 1908 through the school health service and screening is still an important part of the work of the school health worker. Increasingly however the practice of routine medical examination at intervals throughout the child's school life is being replaced by a medical examination at entry and by selective examinations of those children thought to need them thereafter. This screening process is not only directed at specific disease detection but is intended to monitor the child's total health development.

Screening has subsequently been proposed as a means of secondary prevention of a variety of conditions and applicable to all ages – from the very young, even the unborn, to the elderly. It has long been practiced in pregnancy as part of routine ante-natal care while screening the new-born for phenylketonuria and congenital dislocation of the hip are well established. Defects of hearing and of vision can be detected by screening in infancy. The use of mass miniature radiography and cyto-testing has already been referred to. Other conditions for which screening has been used in adults are hypertension, diabetes, cancer of the bladder, of the stomach, and of the lung, mental illness, and glaucoma. The value of screening in the sense of being able to influence the outcome in the patient's favour, has not however been clearly established in most of these conditions.

We shall now consider the case for population screening for breast cancer, as an example chosen because of the considerable public interest in it and because it illustrates some of the problems involved.

Screening for breast cancer
Breast cancer in 1970, the latest year for which complete information is available, was responsible in Great Britain for 19,168 new cases registered, 11,775 deaths, 30,871 hospital admissions and 1,525 hospital beds in continuous use. About one in twenty of young women, should they live long enough, will develop the disease; and about one in 30 of all women will die from it.

The death rate has shown no sign of declining over the past 20 or 30 years; indeed between the ages of 50 and 64 years, the female death rate has risen slightly. There can be no question therefore as to the gravity of the problem; and since we do not know how to prevent breast cancer, the issue whether to institute population screening turns on whether early detection can reduce mortality, and if so by how much and at what cost. The screening procedures available at the present time are clinical examination (palpation) and X-ray of the breast (mammography). In the only extensive trial reported to date (the Health Insurance Plan trial in the USA) it was shown that there were one third fewer deaths during the seven year follow-up among the women who had been offered four screening examinations at annual intervals than in a comparable group who were not offered screening. At first sight the reduction in mortality appears impressive, but even in this large scale trial involving some 60,000 subjects the numbers of deaths in the two groups in seven years were small – 70 and 108 respectively.

It would be unwise to conclude on this evidence that several thousand lives would be saved in this country each year if we had a national screening programme. Indeed some analysts have suggested that the overall reduction in mortality to be expected from a programme on strict HIP lines (that is from four screening examinations and no more for every woman) would be small – perhaps only 3%, though this represents some 300 lives. However, a national programme if embarked upon in this country would almost certainly go beyond the HIP total and if continued indefinitely it has been suggested a 10% reduction in deaths might be a realistic and attainable target. To achieve this reduction the screening programme would have to include both palpation and mammography, since about one-quarter of all cases would be missed if either procedure were omitted. At one time there was concern over the risk involved in exposing women repeatedly to the radiation dose of mammography. The size of the risk was uncertain but it was quite possible that the dosages being given at that time might have caused as many breast cancers as were being detected by screening. Improvements in technique have resulted in radiation exposure being now reduced to what many would regard as acceptable levels. Other methods for early detection of breast cancer such as thermography and ultrasonography, which do not involve any radiation hazard, are being developed and may eventually become considered for use on a population scale.

Whether the false positive rate of present techniques is low enough to be acceptable is another matter. Using both screening techniques there will be at least five 'false positives' for every case of cancer detected and as all 'positives' require a surgical procedure (biopsy) and pathological investigation, a substantial additional load would be placed on the surgical and pathology services if a national screening programme was introduced. Nor should we ignore the anxiety and distress of those women who had to undergo what was to prove in their case an unnecessary, if minor, operation. For the individual woman screening for breast cancer would not be a once for all procedure and every woman would be advised to return for examination at regular intervals. Annual screening is usually suggested but even so the onset of breast cancer may be so rapid that a substantial fraction of all cancers would make themselves known in between screening examinations. Some of these would be false negatives, i.e. cases that had been missed by the screening tests. The danger in such cases is that the woman having been falsely reassured may delay seeking advice even when the cancer becomes apparent at a later time.

The American study was able to demonstrate a definite reduction in mortality only among women in their fifties. No benefit was observed among younger women and no significant advantage to women over 60 years of age. Increasing the number of annual examinations might – or might not – improve on this result. The point is important, first, because only 25 per cent of all breast cancers in this country are detected at ages 50–59 years; and second, in deciding whether a screening programme if there were one, should have a restricted age-at-entry. Information about the likely cost of a national screening programme is scanty, but the Departments of Health have instituted studies which should clarify this and other aspects. There are some 9 million women in Britain aged 50 years and over of whom about 3.5 million are aged 50–59 years. Assuming a 60 per cent response rate, a programme of screening at annual intervals would require 5.4 million tests if all women over 50 were eligible or 2.1 million if the programme were confined to women in their fifties. The number or cancers detected would be of the order of 8,000 and 3,000 respectively and the number of biopsies on false positive cases 40,000 and 15,000 per year respectively. This means that a national screening programme using present techniques, even if restricted to women aged 50–59 years, would involve direct additional expenditure of the order of £20–£30 millions per annum.

There is clearly a need to develop more effective and less expensive techniques for secondary prevention in view of the seriousness of the disease and the lack of any prospect for primary prevention. Nineteen out of twenty women even if they live to an advanced age, will not develop breast cancer. Selection of those at higher-than-average risk would reduce the number who should come for screening regularly.

The greatest advance in screening for breast cancer would come from the development of a test which would identify that sub-group of all women who ought to be screened regularly. Research in this direction is proceeding and it may be possible to achieve the objective by means of a relatively simple estimation of hormones in the urine. Meanwhile, since specialist surgeons and radiologists represent the major part of the cost of conventional screening procedures, the possibility is being explored of using specially trained nurses to conduct the clinical examinations and radiographers to read the mammograms. The public response to a programme that relies in large part on non-medical staff also needs to be assessed. Women can be instructed in self-palpation but how much benefit would follow if the procedure were widely practised is at present an open question.

Prenatal diagnosis
The diagnosis of diseases of the mother that might affect the foetus is not new; tests on the blood of the pregnant woman to detect syphilis were in routine use in the 1930s and for rhesus incompatability from the 1940s.

The aim here is to institute treatment that will as far as possible result in the development of a normal healthy child. During the past decade however, rapid advances have been made in techniques to diagnose abnormal conditions of the foetus with the object, where these are serious enough, of considering abortion. In one sense this amounts to prevention since otherwise the outcome would be the birth of a grossly affected individual.

However, the practice differs fundamentally from population screening because prenatal diagnosis is applied to conditions for which there is no treatment whereas population screening, as has been emphasised, is only justified when treatment can be offered. Although the term 'screening' is already being employed in relation to prenatal diagnosis, it must never be overlooked that the only 'treatment' on offer is termination of pregnancy.

Prenatal diagnosis requires fluid to be drawn from the sac surrounding the baby in the womb. Admission to hospital is unnecessary and there is very little risk to the mother. How much risk, if any, there is to the foetus is being intensively studied but the indications are that in competent hands, the risk is minimal. Amniocentesis as the technique is called is best performed when the pregnancy is 14–15 weeks' old; which ensures that sufficient fluid is available for testing, but is not too late to allow termination of the pregnancy if this is decided upon.

The abnormalities to be considered fall into three main groups – of which 1 and 2 are the most important.

1. Gross malformations of the nervous system (anencephaly and spina bifida) affecting approximately 1 in 200 births.
2. Chromosomal abnormalities, eg Down's Syndrome (mongolism) which occurs in approximately 1 in 600 births.
3. Sex-linked abnormalities.

(There are also some rare metabolic disorders, but the numbers involved are too small to justify a national screening programme.)

MALFORMATION OF THE NERVOUS SYSTEM

There can be few more distressing outcomes of a pregnancy than being delivered of an anencephalic child (lack of development of the brain with no chance of survival). This occurs about once in 500 pregnancies. Hardly less disturbing, and about equally frequent, are other gross malformations of the central nervous system such as severe spina bifida and hydrocephalus. Anencephaly and the more severe forms of spina bifida can be diagnosed with a high degree of certainty by the detection of an abnormal protein in the amniotic fluid. The test is a sensitive one and false positives are exceptional but false negatives have been reported, and the less severe forms of spina bifida are not usually detected by this technique. The only firm indication of higher than average risk is a history of a previously affected offspring, when the probability of gross malformation in a subsequent pregnancy may be as high as 1 in 20. A pregnant women giving such a history should be offered the chance of an amniocentesis.

But this kind of history will represent only 10 per cent of all pregnancies resulting in neural tube (central nervous system) defects and the prospect of monitoring all pregnancies in order to discover the remaining 90 per cent is a daunting one. Fortunately a promising recent development has been the detection at an early stage in affected pregnancies of high levels of the abnormal protein in the mothers' blood serum. It may soon be possible to undertake routinely tests on the mothers' blood in order to select those women who should be offered an amniocentesis.

There are also regional differences in incidence and pilot schemes for large-scale 'pre-screening' by serum tests, already undertaken in parts of Scotland, might also be undertaken in Wales and Northern Ireland where neural tube defects are also known to occur more frequently than elsewhere.

DOWN'S SYNDROME

The position as regards Down's Syndrome (mongolism) is that there are two well-recognised high risk groups; the woman of any age who has already borne an affected offspring and the older pregnant woman irrespective of her previous history. The former group should have any subsequent pregnancies monitored but these women will account for only a small proportion (about 5%) of all cases of Down's Syndrome. The probability of a pregnancy resulting in a live-born affected infant rises rapidly from about 1 in 1,000 for women under the age of 30 years to about 1 in 60 for women of 45 years or older. Since many more babies are born to young mothers, than to older women, most affected infants are also born to young mothers, the maternal-age effect notwithstanding. Thus, monitoring all pregnancies where the mother was, say, aged 40 years and over, with termination of all positives, would have reduced the number of live-born mongol children in England and Wales in 1973 by 14%.

SEX-LINKED DISORDERS

It is relatively easy to determine the sex of the foetus from a sample obtained by amniocentesis, and termination of pregnancy can be considered where there is a risk of sex-linked disorders such as haemophilia or one particular type of muscular dystrophy. In these disorders the

F

female 'carries' the abnormal gene but only males are affected. The usual reason for monitoring the pregnancy in such cases will be the birth of an earlier affected male infant. Less often a well-documented family history will have suggested that an amniocentesis might be advisable. If a pregnant woman is known to be (because she has already given birth to an affected offspring), or suspected (from the family history) of being a carrier, the sex of the foetus can be determined. If a female, the infant would not be affected (but would have a 50:50 chance of being a carrier) whereas if a male, there is a 50:50 chance of its being affected. There are no means at present of diagnosing these disorders in the foetus, only of establishing the sex and thus the probability of its being affected. Nevertheless, the parents, if they have already had experience of an affected child may wish to consider termination (in the event of the foetus being male) even though there is an even chance that a normal foetus would be aborted.

Some general considerations

The incidence in future generations of the abnormalities for which pre-natal diagnosis is proposed will not be appreciably reduced by eliminating affected foetuses in this generation. In other words, a programme of prenatal diagnosis and termination of affected pregnancies is not self-limiting; once started it must go on until the 'causes' of abnormalities are discovered and removed.

The cost aspects of prenatal diagnosis are referred to in Chapter VII (page 86). It would be quite impracticable to apply these techniques to all pregnancies if only because the expert staff to deal with 800,000 procedures a year does not exist and it would take several years to recruit and train them in sufficient numbers. Selective screening on the other hand is likely to be practised on an increasing scale in the fore-seeable future.

There is however an additional dimension to many aspects of prenatal diagnosis and the possible steps which follow from it – namely the ethical issues. While such issues occur in many aspects of medical care they are in this area particularly pointed and open to argument.

For many of the abnormalities being considered, eg Down's Syndrome, there is no cure; and the choice lies between abortion or the birth of an affected individual. How should the community weigh the interests of an individual yet unborn? Sometimes the parents will have already had experience of the disease eg muscular dystrophy; in such cases should their wishes be accepted as paramount? For yet other conditions, eg haemophilia, the choice lies between termination of pregnancy, when half the males aborted would have been normal, and protracted and expensive treatment, the cost of which in one form or another would fall on the community, possibly to the exclusion of treatment or care for some other group. Many children with Down's Syndrome now survive to adult life and again the cost of their care over many years may have to be borne by the community. One group where the problem does not arise in this form is anencephalic children, who from the nature of their condition have no chance of survival beyond birth.

Some would argue that it is the right and duty of the community to provide full facilities for 'selective termination of pregnancy' which parents can use if they wish where there is good evidence of the likely abnormality of the foetus. Others would argue against this and would say that the community and parents should accept the responsibility of caring for all children, however severely handicapped at birth. Detailed examination of these ethical considerations must lie outside the scope of this paper but deciding how the resources of the community can best be spent among the competing claims of various groups, each with their own problems, takes us into the question of costs, benefits and resources discussed in the next chapter.

CHAPTER VII Costs, benefits and resources

Introduction

All over the world there has been an explosive growth in the cost of medical care and Britain is by no means the country worst affected. The impact has been such that the cost effectiveness of medical procedures is being questioned more closely than ever before.

Medical care is, quite apart from the ever increasing cost of sophisticated equipment, also labour intensive. An essential part of the service is the personal relationship between patient and doctor, nurse or other health professional. It is impossible to put a price tag on such a relationship but it would be both difficult and foolish to attempt to economise too much on it.

As medical science progresses new techniques and new possibilities are thrown up which creates tension between what is technically possible and what our resources – especially at a time of economic restraint – can sustain. Nor is this tension produced only by technical progress. It often arises from what one might almost call a moral change. We wish, for example, to improve the conditions of the mentally handicapped. Here too, science may intervene by raising their life expectancy and hence their numbers and increasing the costs involved.

Prevention is better than cure – but is it also cheaper? This is not always an easy question to answer. Where, by relatively inexpensive means we can avoid condemning someone to a lifetime of physical dependence the answer will almost certainly be 'yes' – often because there is no cure. But it would be foolish not to recognise that there may also be cases where the advantages of prevention must be purchased at the cost of other services. Nor must we forget the paradox that prevention (or cure, for that matter) by enabling more people to reach an age at which they are increasingly likely to become dependent may eventually increase the calls on our national resources.

Vaccination and immunisation/poliomyelitis

One preventive procedure where it can be confidently asserted that cost savings are apparent and substantial is poliomyelitis immunisation.

The economic attractiveness of vaccination and immunisation programmes depends upon three factors, apart from the cost of the vaccine. These are the risk of getting the disease; how difficult it is to treat and cure; and the extent to which the vaccine has side effects. The poliomyelities immunisation programme has been successful according to these criteria. In particular the high cost of treating the disease and its effects in terms of physical handicap and premature death imply very large financial benefits in addition to the human benefits in terms of reduced suffering, longer life and so on. The overall financial benefits of a poliomyelitis programme over twenty years in terms of savings in medical costs and the productivity of those who avoided the disease have been estimated at twelve times the cost of the immunisation. Poliomyelitis vaccination is one example of measures in which, even if humanitarian considerations were completely absent, rational economic calculation would suggest that vigorous action be taken.

Fluoridation

A good example of a programme which could save money is fluoridation of water supplies. The cost would, on average, amount to no more than a few pence per annum per head. The prevalence of dental caries would be reduced by an average of 50%, or possibly more if fluoridation is combined with other dental hygiene procedures, and the average reduction would be greater as the exposure of the population increased over time.

But would fluoridation actually save money? Possibly not, in a strictly financial sense. A large part of the 'savings' will accrue in the form of improved dental care. In the longer run also, those whose natural teeth have been saved by fluoridation will require further dental care; but so, to some extent, would those who have lost their teeth at an early age. Nevertheless, a successful fluoridation campaign should improve dental health and also make it possible to transfer some resources to other forms of dental care and to other sectors.

Road accidents

Another area where financial savings can be clearly seen is in reducing the number of road accidents. It has been estimated that such accidents cost the health service about £40 million a year. The value of lost output attributable to them is some £215 million, the damage to property about £135 million, and the costs of police and administration come to another £25 million.

It has also been estimated that the universal use of seat belts would reduce the number of fatal and serious injuries by between 15% and 20% with consequent savings of some £50 million a year. If the initial success of the breath test in reducing accidents had been maintained the likely savings would have amounted to about £45 million a year.

Screening and prenatal diagnosis

The possibility of detecting disease at an early stage by the use of a cheap easily-administered screening procedure is an attractive one. Where such procedures can economise on the use of scarce skilled staff then their advantages would seem even more evident.

But some caution is necessary. No matter how cheap a test is, it is still expensive if it does not lead to a significant number of cases of a disease for which there is an effective treatment being discovered. A relatively cheap method now exists for screening young girls for bacteriuria (the presence of abnormal quantities of bacteria in the urine). The test can be largely self-administered, its cost is little more than 30p a head, and it costs about £15 on average to discover a case. So far, however, there is little or no evidence that the condition has any long-term clinical significance, and if this is so, money spent on discovering it is money wasted.

Even where a test does pick up cases of a treatable disease in its early stages this in itself is still not enough to justify the expenditure on it. One of the earliest population screening programmes was the mass X-ray campaign principally directed at the detection of tuberculosis. As the disease became less common the cost per case found rose. At the same time drug treatment had improved and became increasingly effective irrespective of the stage of the disease. On balance it probably became more expensive to pick up cases of the disease early by indiscriminate screening since in addition some might have cured themselves naturally. Whether the benefits from completely eliminating the disease would be great enough to offset the costs would depend on several factors, one being the effectiveness of the method used for case detection.

Many similar problems are raised by breast cancer screening. The average cost of screening a woman for breast cancer is about £6 a time – the cost per life prolonged probably about £8,000 although a selective programme might be able, for a lower total yield, to reduce this to £2,000 to £3,000 at which price perhaps as much as 10% of the number of deaths from breast cancer could be saved in the long-run.

When resources are limited, there is an unanswerable case for concentrating them where they can do most good. The procedure for detecting Down's Syndrome (mongolism) is a comparatively expensive one because it involves a rather labour-intensive laboratory procedure (See Chapter VI). The current cost of the test is about £80 per head. The risk of the condition increases sharply with the age of the mother so that the cost of detecting the presence of every affected foetus is less than £8,000 for mothers aged 40 or over but might be £80,000 for mothers under 30 years of age.

Apart from the medical conditions to which they are prone in infancy and childhood, mongol children may require, as many do, eventually to be cared for in institutions imposing a further heavy burden on the health service. Improved medical care now ensures that many more of the children survive infancy – perhaps as many as 80 per cent. Therefore although the number of mongol births has been declining, the number of those affected who are alive is probably increasing. It costs about £2,000 a year to keep somebody in a mental handicap hospital and the cost of special education is about £1,000 a year. These sorts of costs which would be avoided if there were fewer mongol births must be set against the cost of the programme itself. It seems likely that for mothers aged, say, 40 and over the costs to society of caring for the affected children and adults would in total exceed the cost of a screening programme. For younger mothers the risk of affected infants and the economic advantage of screening is less certain. A comprehensive programme for all mothers would be impossible to implement in the short run in any case because of the vast demands it would make on medical and technical staff.

The maternal blood test for severe spina bifida, referred to in Chapter VI, probably costs less than £3 a head. Since the risk of the condition varies greatly according to geographical region the cost of detecting a foetus with spina bifida might range from £1,000 to £4,000. The test also detects the presence of anencephaly but this condition does not have the long-term consequences of spina bifida. The grossly handicapped spina bifida child and adult makes large demands on the health and social services. It seems likely that, in general, the cost of these demands will exceed the cost of a programme to detect the condition.

Health education

There is much potential for prevention in health education aimed at altering people's attitudes towards such things as tobacco, alcohol and exercise – persuading them in effect to invest in their own health. Government can play a role by altering the structure of incentives facing people, by reducing the cost of, for example, investing in physical recreation or by acquiring information about the dangers of cigarette smoking through health education, but the onus of making the decisions in order to safeguard health must necessarily rest on the individual. The Health

Education Council, which was set up by the then Government in 1968, has major responsibilities at national level in England, Wales and Northern Ireland for the promotion and development of health education. In Scotland similar functions are carried out by the Scottish Health Education Unit and the Scottish Council for Health Education. The Government intends to continue to give full support to these bodies.

Discussion

Cynics often say, particularly in regard to smoking, that prevention is not worth the effort; that it will only lead to greater expense, because those who do not die early live to reach the age of dependence when they must be supported from public funds and eventually die of some other disease which may necessitate medical care at public expense. Quite apart from the fact that prevention is valuable even if it is expensive, the argument has other weaknesses. Firstly, much prevention will serve to increase the active earning life of individuals rather than simply to avert premature death. This reduces the demand on public funds. Secondly, even if prevention only postponed the costs of medical care, postponing costs has an economic value which can be quite substantial.

The problem of who shall benefit from preventive measures also raises difficulties. As has been stressed earlier, for many diseases there are groups of the population which are at higher risk than others. If value for money were the sole consideration one might wish to restrict preventive and screening programmes to these high risk groups which will give the greatest yield for a given expenditure of money. But this aim may conflict with the principle that everyone should have equal access to medical care if they can possibly benefit from it. And yet if everyone is to have equal access to medical care and the funds available are limited then the number of preventive programmes which can be carried on will be less and the amount of avoidable illness or premature death will be greater. There is no easy solution to this dilemma and the balance which will be struck is bound to be one which will not satisfy everybody.

It has been claimed that the next important step forward in preventive medicine would be the prevention of stroke by the control of high blood pressure and no single advance, possibly, would do more to enhance the quality of life. Cerebrovascular disease is one of the commonest causes of hospital admission (over 110,000 admissions a year in Great Britain) and one of the greatest 'consumers' of hospital beds (about 20,000 beds occupied every day) and in addition there are an unknown number of patients cared for at home, in local authority accommodation and in nursing homes. Population screening for high blood pressure is probably feasible and drugs are available to control mild degrees of hypertension. What has yet to be established is whether large numbers of people in their middle years would be prepared to take the drugs regularly for the rest of their lives and whether, even if they did, the incidence of stroke would be significantly reduced. But assuming both questions were answered in the affirmative, the decision would then have to be faced, could the cost of the programme, running perhaps into several tens of millions a year, be met? This example ought not to be regarded as exceptional.

The cost of fitting all motor cars with filters to reduce the emission of lead in exhaust fumes had been estimated at £1,000 million and the benefits to be expected are, according to some experts, uncertain. No generally agreed estimates have been compiled of what it cost the country to implement the Clean Air Act 1956 and we can only guess at the size of the health benefits.

Whilst there is clearly plenty of scope for preventive action involving substantial expenditure, there are also many possibilities for the introduction of measures which do not necessarily require additional or substantial financial resources.

In this connection the important contribution to prevention which the individual can make for himself should be emphasised. To follow the recommended schedule of vaccination and immunisation usually involves no more than visiting the nearest health centre or clinic. Many smokers pay dearly in hard cash for indulging their habit and so too do people who drink to excess. It costs nothing to fasten a seat-belt once provided and reckless driving can be a very expensive way of getting to one's destination – or of not getting there. Taking regular exercise need not involve substantial expenditure for the individual. Facilities for swimming, one of the best forms of exercise, are being brought within reach of more and more people and the cost of walking is measured in shoe-leather. There is a danger that people are led to think they have discharged their responsibility for their own health if they have taken this test or accepted that procedure. Important though these are, there is more to it than that.

This chapter began by noting that the expense of medical care is growing rapidly. A week in a typical hospital now costs, on average, nearly £150. If prevention programmes can avoid or postpone costs of this order then they can contribute mightily to a higher standard of care for those who are unavoidably ill. Where preventive programmes must compete for scarce funds with other programmes it is more than ever necessary that decisions should be taken in the fullest possible knowledge of all the factors involved.

CHAPTER VIII Retrospect and prospect

Lessons from experience

As shown in the early chapters, the enormous advances in public health during the last century have led to a doubling of the population despite a halving of the birthrate. During the second half of this period, while the expectation of life at early ages has continued to lengthen, the improvement at later ages has been much less – especially for men.

The chief lesson of this historical review is the complexity of the reasons for improvements in health. Some diseases have declined for reasons which are still quite obscure. But only to a limited extent and in comparatively recent times can these improvements be clearly attributed to strictly medical activities, such as immunisation or the use of antibiotics. Over the longer term they owe much more to better nutrition, better housing, sanitary engineering, higher standards of personal hygiene and to other wider social and economic changes.

This complexity offers opportunities for intervention at many different points in the natural history of a disease process. Though we no longer have malaria in these islands except when, as is increasingly common, travellers bring it in, it is a clear example of this principle. To prevent malaria, we can drain the marshes where disease carrying mosquitoes breed, kill the mosquitoes with insecticides or take anti-malarial tablets to prevent the growth of the malaria organism after it has been conveyed by mosquito bites.

Given a choice of strategies, which is the strategy of choice? This will vary with the circumstances. In a given situation some strategies may be more effective than others and some may be cheaper. Depending on the choice, the key person to combat malaria may be the civil engineer, the man with the spray gun, or the home visitor who distributes the anti-malarial medicine. But others too, will be involved; the epidemiologist who knows about mosquitoes, the chemist who developed the non-toxic anti-malarial drug; the economist who can estimate the balance of cost and benefit; the health educator who helps to secure public understanding and co-operation; and government authorities must ultimately decide which strategy to adopt and find the necessary funds. Nor must we forget the ordinary man, woman and child, on whom ultimately the success of the third strategy will depend. There is nothing unique about this example – if there is any field which is demonstrably 'multi-disciplinary', it is the prevention of disease.

Another lesson to be learned from history is that even incomplete knowledge may be adequate for the purpose of preventive action. As was pointed out in Chapter II with respect to cholera, skin cancer and scurvy, a considerable time elapsed between finding effective ways of prevention and discovering the specific causes of these diseases. These examples, taken from such diverse fields as infectious disease, cancer and nutritional deficiency, serve to emphasise how general is this principle of the adequacy of incomplete knowledge. But knowledge is not enough, since its possession is no guarantee that it will always be applied. These examples serve to illustrate this elementary but sometimes overlooked truth. Epidemics of cholera still occur where water supplies are liable to faecal pollution; Captain Scott's Antarctic expedition came to grief largely because of scurvy due to deficiency in the rations; and cases of chemically induced skin cancer still arise in this country.

We can also see from history how easy it can be to draw unwarranted conclusions about the real causes of change. The death rate from whooping cough, to take one example, dropped in the 40 years from 1895 to 1935 by about 80%. No doubt there were those during that period who were ready enough to claim the credit for one nostrum or other, but we know now that specific treatment either for the disease or for its complications was not in fact available until the late 1930s.

Chapter III outlined the health problems facing Western society today, setting the scene for the remainder of our survey of disease prevention. An examination of the statistics of disease and of the changes in our social and physical environment indicate the four main groups of health problems which face us today; those concerned with the ageing of the populaion, with an unhealthy life-style, with mental health, and with environmental hazards. But the fact that such problems are looming large does not mean that we can stand down our traditional defences, based on such well-tried measures as immunisation and the control of food hygiene.

Finally, history shows that with sufficient determination many health problems are solved. The fall in maternal mortality was due to concerted and sustained effort by Goverment, both central and local and by the health professions (including administrators and statisticians who are not normally classed as health professionals).

Chapter IV posed challenges for everyone concerned with the provision of health services. Major differences in statistical indices between countries, between regions, and between social classes suggest the enormous potential scope for prevention. All those concerned with the health services should ask how their local statistics compare with other areas, regions and nations; and when differences are found to occur – as they certainly will – they should ask themselves and their professional advisers these questions. Why do these differences exist? Where the causes are known, can they be removed? If so, how? Is there something the health authority itself can do, or is some other authority or organisation better placed to take action? Just as causes are complex so remedies are rarely simple, and often the disparities revealed in statistical comparisons raise wide-ranging issues of social and economic policy.

Infant mortality is often regarded as the traditional index of the efficiency of the preventive services. The situation revealed in Chapter IV leaves no room for complacency, and improvements in our preventive programmes are undoubtedly possible. For example, deaths and disability from haemolytic disease of the new-born still occur; but they are almost entirely avoidable, if the system which has been devised functions smoothly. Congenital defects resulting from rubella (german measles) during pregnancy should be entirely avoidable if the preventive system is working well.

The key to prevention is often the identification of 'risk factors' and thus of 'vulnerable groups'. A risk factor is a characteristic of an individual which has been found to be statistically associated with a disease. Where such an association is known to exist between a characteristic and a disease, the persons possessing this characteristic are a vulnerable group. They have a higher than average risk of the disease. The association does not of necessity imply that the mechanism of causation has been found, but it will nevertheless indicate the target group at which preventive action should be aimed. We know that 9 out of 10 people who develop lung cancer are or have been cigarette smokers. Cigarette smokers are at risk of lung cancer and should be persuaded to give up smoking. We know that mothers who first attend antenatal clinics late in pregnancy and parents who do not use the child care services are vulnerable groups. Of course not all their offspring will come to harm but a disproportionate number will do so. These are the families that should be given particular attention in any programme of prevention.

Chapter V discussed problems arising from people's life-styles. This raises complex issues of the apportionment of responsibility between the individual, society as a whole and government. Some would put the emphasis on the role of the individual who should refrain from cigarette smoking, excessive self-indulgence and other behaviour which places his health at risk. Others would say that government should either impose more control or do more to educate and persuade the public – or both. Yet others blame the way society is organised and the stresses that this imposes on individuals – even though, for example, countries with high alcoholism rates are as varied in their social and political structure as are countries with low rates. How far should the individual be free to harm himself, when society has to deal with the consequences? Now that motorcyclists are compelled to wear crash helmets, should motorists be compelled to wear seat belts?

Chapter v went on to discuss the dilemmas of uncertainty. Decisions have to be taken on the prevention of disease even though we cannot be sure of the relevance or validity of the available evidence. Inaction is just as much a decision as action. How does one balance an unknown risk against a known advantage? The same question frequently arises in the actual practice of medicine. The growing complexity of medical investigation and treatment has increased the risk of disease and injury resulting from the actions of doctors, nurses, and technicians. In 1972 about 100,000 hospital admissions in England and Wales were caused by the adverse effects of medicines and the complications of surgical procedures and medical care. Nor is this a new problem; medical and social policies pursued in the past led to the 'institutionalisation' of the mentally ill, the mentally handicapped, the elderly and the disabled in ways which all too often accentuated rather than relieved that individual problem. It was Florence Nightingale who wrote in 1863 that 'it may seem a strange principle as the very first requirement in a hospital that it should do the sick no harm'.

Chapter vi explained the meaning of 'screening' and discussed the reasons for adopting, or deciding not to adopt, a particular form of it. Prenatal diagnosis is a major technical advance which will become increasingly important in future but it poses ethical issues of great difficulty. It is society as a whole and not simply Government or the health professions alone that will have to try to resolve these questions.

The theme of Chapter vii was that the costs of preventive measures should be related to the benefits they are expected to bring. Effectiveness (does the measure work?) needs to be related to efficiency (at what cost – in terms of money, manpower, and material resources?). Prevention does not necessarily involve extra resources: it may be that existing resources can be better used or diverted to a different purpose. In the early years of the National Health Service there was an acute shortage of maternity beds and even those that were available were inefficiently used from the point of view of maternal safety. Increasingly hospital beds were allocated to mothers-to-be on the basis of risk. This undoubtedly helped to reduce maternal and peri-natal mortality until more beds could be provided and selection became unnecessary. There is always a need to concentrate resources where they can do most good. We are currently trying to predict more accurately infants most at risk of sudden and unexpected death ('cot deaths') and of non-accidental injury ('baby battering') so that preventive services can be especially channelled to these families. Because circumstances change and knowledge grows, preventive programmes must be constantly re-examined to see if they are still both effective and efficient in using resources. For what was soundly-based routine practice yesterday may become a waste of resources tomorrow.

This means that new knowledge must be translated into practice as soon as possible and that enough resources must be spent on expanding knowledge through research. Research can help to unravel the causes of variations in health standards such as those set out in Chapter IV. This is the traditional task of epidemiology which should increasingly seek those causes of disease which can be eliminated or reduced. Secondly, research is needed to find more effective ways of delivering preventive care. How can we increase the numbers of people who are immunised? How effective are health advisory services for young people? What is the best form of public education to tackle a particular health problem? Finally, research is needed to find more efficient ways of preventing disease.

Most plans to prevent disease depend on health education of the public. One reason why maternity beds were used inefficiently twenty and more years 'ago was because many women did not understand the benefits of going into hospital to have their baby. To a large extent, the success of a screening programme depends on finding the people who are most at risk and persuading them to take part. Health education as practised by midwives, health visitors and school nurses has in the past been enormously successful in improving the health of mothers and children, and in promoting vaccination and immunisation programmes. New initiatives in health education are now needed to tackle, for example, child abuse and to help and prepare individuals and families to meet the pressures of living in modern society.

Taking it on from here
This summary and indeed this paper make no claims to be comprehensive. It is intended to encourage others to extend the work and fill in the gaps. It is a consultative paper which deliberately poses more questions

than it answers. None of the major health issues mentioned have been examined in depth and no specific programme of action is recommended. The united action which it is intended to stimulate is discussion by laymen as well as professionals and what we should ourselves be doing to improve the quality of our own lives and the lives of others. Prevention is not just a matter for action or discussion by experts, it concerns us all. Most of us can improve our own health and that of the community.

The health authorities and the Community and Local Health Councils have a special responsibility for developing the preventive aspects of their work. The fact that resources are under pressure makes it that much more important to see that what is available is used as effectively as possible. Health Authorities will wish to consider, in the light of this paper, whether and how their policies should be orientated more towards prevention – if necessary at the cost of something else. Increased attention to prevention may in the long run release resources by reducing the numbers needing cure and care so that better cure and care can be provided for those whose conditions are harder to prevent or more difficult to postpone.

Doctors, nurses and health visitors and many others can advise and help individuals to help themselves. For a recurring theme of this paper is how much, today, prevention depends on the attitude of the individual to his own life style. People do respond to advice from those they respect.

Members of local authorities and those working for them with responsibilities for the social services, environmental health, and the education services, have all an important part to play in the preservation and development of community health standards. Also voluntary bodies have, as mentioned in Chapter I, often shown the way in preventive work and are still breaking new ground. For example, the WRVS developed the meals-on-wheels service. Many voluntary services help maintain sanity and morale in the face of sudden or severe tribulation. The churches have long practised pastoral work of this nature. More recently Alcoholics Anonymous and the Samaritans have provided services of this kind in a new form.

Much of the responsibility for ensuring his own good health lies with the individual. We can all influence others by our own actions. In particular, parents can set their children a good example of healthy living. We can all help to influence the communities in which we live and work as much by our example as by our efforts.

In central government, the Health Departments can set standards, spread ideas, finance health education, provide technical support and sponsor research. But prevention is also the concern directly or indirectly of other

Government Departments such as the Department of the Environment, (environmental health), the Department of Employment and the Health and Safety Commission (occupational health), the Ministry of Agriculture, Fisheries and Food (food standards) and the Department of Education and Science (the teaching of health) – with the Scottish Office, the Welsh Office, and the Northern Ireland Office, playing a key role over several of these areas together in the different parts of the United Kingdom.

The first aim of this paper is, therefore, to promote discussion and the Health Departments will welcome comments on this paper. But it will have failed in its purpose if this discussion does not lead in turn to positive action to promote health

- action which individuals take in relation to the health and well being of themselves and their family.
- action in planning and reorienting local and national services to give a greater emphasis to prevention within whatever resources can be made available.

Finally, as indicated in the opening chapter, the Government will follow up this paper over the next few years by publishing a series of more detailed papers on specific aspects of prevention. The momentum will be maintained. Prevention is the key to healthier living and a higher quality of life for all of us.

Printed in England for Her Majesty's Stationery Office
By Tonbridge Printers Ltd,
Shipbourne Road, Tonbridge, Kent
Dd 290600 K540 2/76